# SECRETS FROM A
# HERBALIST'S
# GARDEN

## JO DUNBAR

ILLUSTRATED BY THE INK HERMIT

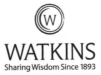

## WATKINS
Sharing Wisdom Since 1893

I would really like to thank Adam Gordon for making this book possible, for without you, I know it wouldn't be. My thanks too to The Ink Hermit, a beautiful soul, whose drawings are so sublime and perfectly reflect my impressions of the delicate nature of plants. And I would like to thank my partner Adrian Rooke for his support and enthusiasm in helping me to collect my herbs, press the tinctures and talk through aspects of this book. The retreats which we have run together over the years have given much inspiration for this book.

**Secrets from a Herbalist's Garden**

Jo Dunbar

First published in the UK and USA in 2022 by Watkins, an imprint of Watkins Media Limited Unit 11, Shepperton House, 83–93 Shepperton Road London N1 3DF

enquiries@watkinspublishing.com

**Commissioning Editor:** Adam Gordon
**Editor:** Hayley Shepherd
**Managing Designer:** Karen Smith
**Designer:** Alice Claire Coleman
**Production:** Uzma Taj

A CIP record for this book is available from the British Library

ISBN: 978-1-78678-662-3 (Paperback)
ISBN: 978-1-78678-703-3 (eBook)

10 9 8 7 6 5 4 3 2 1

Typeset in Cera Pro
Printed in the UK by TJ Books

**Publisher's note:**

www.watkinspublishing.com

**Note:**

Do not mix metric, imperial and US cup measurements: 1 tsp = 5ml, 1 tbsp = 15ml, 1 cup = 240ml

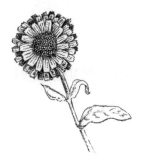

FOR THE ANCIENT ONES,
EVER YOUNG

# CONTENTS

# INTRODUCTION

Breathing hard as I climb the steep side of the wooded slope, it is a relief to reach the contour path, and catch my breath as I walk under the yew boughs. Prisms of sunlight piercing the dark forest, light captured in spider's webs, I walk silently on soft needle-covered clay, then through a tunnel of prickly brambles with wild roses catching on my clothes, and suddenly, I burst, blinking, out of the forest and into the sunlight, high up in the hills.

Up here are ancient meadows, yellow with St John's wort, sweet-smelling lady's bedstraw, lofty agrimony and wispy dandelions. Mounds of wild purple thyme, the hot summer air fragrant with *origanum*. Flying creatures whip past my ears as wild roses tear at my jeans and spiders creep under my shirt. Lonely winds blow, butterflies spiral around each other, birds cry and the ghosts of ancient chiefs buried in the tumuli above watch me perform the other oldest profession in the world: gathering herbs for medicine.

Down from the hills and back in the village which I call home is my herb garden, alive with birds, a few voles, a grass snake and raised beds of herbs. A small kitchen is hung with more herbs, scented with boiling berries and the sharp tang of thyme. I am making medicine for the winter.

There is no greater alchemy than collecting healing plants from your garden or the wild, transforming them into medicine through a simple method of extraction, giving that medicine to someone in need and letting the herbs do their healing work by the grace of Mother Nature.

The entire process is magical: the collecting, alone amongst the hills on warm sunny days with only the buzzards swirling above in clear azure skies as your witness. Here I walk, high on the hills above a flock of swifts, where the lonely winds blow with echoes of past herbalists doing the same as I am now. Even on cold, bracing days with a wild wind battering your face, or gently caressing your garden plants as you harvest them – it is almost ethereal, like stepping into another dimension.

Then the hammering of conkers, shaving of roots, chopping of soft herbage, the stirring, boiling, straining, and finally – the healing. It is a beautiful way of life. Much forgotten, but now a great remembering is stirring. People want to reconnect with the land again. They want to tap into the wisdom of it, and they want to use plants in their homes for medicine.

Herbal medicine is traditionally women's work. Although there have been plenty of excellent and famous male herbalists, by and large, it has always been women's work. They used what was available. Not that long ago, doctors were far too expensive for most folk, plus their medicine was as likely to kill as to cure. Like organic farming, plants do not dominate the body, but work with it to restore health. The plants which grow on these lands have powerful healing qualities and are perfectly disposed to being used for home herbal remedies. This is how the women of old would heal – not with expensive exotic herbs, but just the plants which they grew in their gardens, which grew in the fields, and we can do the same. They also used some rather gruesome and bizarre recipes, but we won't go into snail-oil cough mixture or earthworm love potions here.

This is a book of plant remedies, born of over 22 years of my personal experience as a medical herbalist. I have chosen to write only about herbs which you can either grow or collect, or find in your kitchen cupboard, and so we save air miles, carbon and money. These remedies work.

# CHAPTER 1

## The Winter Solstice

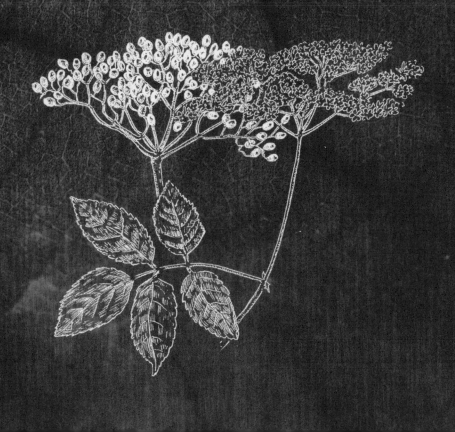

The silence of the Winter Solstice. A time when the sun appears to pause, as if taking a great shuddering breath before its apparent rebirth. For us down here on this beautiful planet, it is as if the Earth Mother stops to listen for a call from somewhere far away in the darkness of our solar system. A cry from the Sun Child, for on the Winter Solstice, the Sun God is reborn. All over Europe and the British Isles lie ancient monuments marking this great time of the year. Stonehenge, Newgrange, Maeshowe – all honouring the rebirth of the Sun God.

People have gathered for thousands of years at these and other monuments on solstice morning, to witness the sun piercing the darkness, penetrating the Earth. At solstice sunrise, a light is ignited in the dark half of the year, and the waltz of the seasons strikes up once again as we begin our stately dance through the turning of the year. Out of the darkest days, the sun will very slowly begin to grow in strength once again. Without that light, all life ceases.

On the edge of the forested hill opposite my home grows a beautiful beech tree. The leaves of this tree form a face, and I call him my Green Man. Every day I look out the window and have a little chat, and I have even fancied that I can divine what my day will be like by the expression on his face. For the most part, he is jolly, but sometimes he looks worried. In the late autumn, I notice that as the leaves start falling, his face turns upside down as if he is diving back into the Earth for the winter.

So, it is thus that the energies of the plants descend deep down into the Earth Mother, where they lie quietly, resting and recuperating from the busyness of the growing season. Over the winter, within the dark nourishment of the earth, they gather their resources for the spring to come. So too should we.

Now, in our own lives, we can withdraw into the quiet of the dark nights, and take out some of the herbs which we have gathered and stored over the past year, to make the tonics and potions which are going to keep us strong throughout the cold, dark months. On a winter's night, I love to close my curtains against the black winds and rain, light a fire, and start brewing and stewing in my kitchen.

# IMMUNITY, COLDS AND FLU

🌿 ELDERBERRIES 🌿 TURMERIC 🌿 OLIVE
🌿 GARLIC 🌿 BLACKBERRIES 🌿 LEMON BALM 🌿 SAGE
🌿 ROWAN BERRY 🌿 HORSERADISH 🌿 ELECAMPANE
🌿 ONIONS 🌿 WILD GARLIC 🌿 JACK-BY-THE-HEDGE
🌿 THYME 🌿 GOOSEGRASS 🌿 ANGELICA
🌿 WILD LETTUCE 🌿 SLOES

Early December is only the beginning of winter. Although we still carry the warmth and strength from summer, by the end of a long year, already, our inner resources are fading. Now we need to boost up our immune systems and keep them strong in preparation for the coming cold, dark months.

At this time, our resources are outside of our bodies, in the form of herbs which we have harvested, or swapped with our friends, or if necessary, purchased. All of these are common herbs and spices and are easily available to everybody. They are also very safe, and very effective.

After over 22 years as a medical herbalist, I have come to the opinion that there are two aspects of our lives which form the foundation of robust health, and those are good food and a good mood. So, bearing in mind Hippocrates, who advised us to "Let food be thy medicine and medicine be thy food", I often consider what our grandmothers might have cooked during the dark cold months. Well, it certainly wasn't hummus and avocado salads. At this time of year, they would have been stirring hearty pottages, made with chicken stock (great for loosening mucus and reducing the inflammation caused by infection) or bone broth with root vegetables full of hearty nourishment. No doubt they would have retrieved from their pantries a handful of immune-boosting dried mushrooms and one or two strong antibacterial onions and garlic, some cabbage from the garden, and possibly added thyme, winter savory or parsley too. All of these ingredients are bursting with nutrients and antibacterial properties.

Assuming you, dear reader, like most modern citizens, are leading a very busy life, possibly teaching a classroom full of children, working in an open office or using public transport to get to and from the office, you cannot help but pick up the various viruses flying around at this time of the year. You are probably feeling cold and weary, with your resources much depleted. Let's consider how you can strengthen yourself and your family.

The first step is to begin by nourishing yourself with a cauldron of chicken soup, or if you are vegan or vegetarian, then leave out the chicken and make a mushroom and root vegetable stock instead as your base.

## COUGHS, COLDS AND FLU

Antibiotics may kill bacteria but not viruses; however, they also kill the trillions of friendly immune-boosting bacteria which live in our intestines. Herbal antibacterials and antivirals do not appear to compromise our gut flora. They are also able to strengthen our immune system to fight the bugs from within.

There are some home remedies which are very effective at boosting our immune system, killing bronchial infections and helping us to feel much better. Some of the herbs, such as elderberries, you would have harvested earlier in the year, and either made into a cordial, or dried and stored, are now ready to turn into something magical! And it is magical. Picking a weed, stirring it into a medicine and then getting well from your remedy was the first magic, and it is empowering to protect and heal your family with what we now call a weed. For what is a weed? Why, it is a plant whose benevolence has been forgotten.

## IMMUNE-BOOSTING SOUP

🌿 Start with 1 organic chicken, slowly simmering in a large saucepan of water.

🌿 Add to the water 2 strong onions, some organic celery and carrots, immune-boosting shiitake mushrooms, grated fresh turmeric (which is famous for its anti-inflammatory properties), a handful of antibacterial thyme and a few cloves of garlic.

🌿 Cover the pot and simmer for about 2 hours, then switch off the heat but leave the lid on, and leave overnight. In the morning, you should have a jelly-like collagen-rich stock to work with.

🌿 Carefully lift out the chicken; pull off the meat, throw away the bones and give the skins to the dogs, cats or foxes.

🌿 Strain the stock, and then you can add the root vegetables of your choice. Personally, I love to add potatoes and butternut squash, or legumes such as brown lentils or kidney beans, and some leeks and mushrooms for flavour.

🌿 Cook these vegetables in your stock until they are soft, then either blend smooth or leave as is for a chunky soup. You can return the chicken meat to the soup at this point, if you want to.

🌿 You should now have a lovely thick broth, full of nutrients, which is easy to digest and very comforting. Just before you serve, you might like to add a handful of freshly chopped chives for extra flavour and antibacterial qualities.

*"Let food be thy medicine and medicine be thy food"*

# IMMUNE-BOOSTING HERBS

## Elderberries (*Sambucus nigra*)

The elder tree is one of nature's great medicine chests. It is one of my great joys in late summer to wander down long hedges of elder trees with my lovely partner, Adrian, collecting baskets of the dark juicy berries whilst outraged sheep glower and yell at us for trespassing on their field.

Over and over, I am amazed at the wisdom and generosity of nature. This tree produces flowers at the height of the hay-fever season in May. The blossoms have exceptional anti-inflammatory effects on our mucous membranes, making them excellent for the immediate home treatment of hay fever (see page 133).

By the end of summer, just before the cold and flu season strikes, the flowers swell into clusters of blue-black berries, bursting with vitamin C, as well as having significant antiviral properties!

Elderberries have been used since at least medieval times for the prevention and treatment of colds and flu, but with science, we now have a clearer understanding as to how they work. As an antiviral, elderberry is as clever in its mechanism of protection as the virus's mechanism of attack.

As everyone learned from Covid-19, viruses cannot reproduce themselves, but need to penetrate our cell walls in order to access our genetic RNA. The virus has spikes on its outer membrane, which bind to our own cells, then penetrate our cell walls to gain entry, where it hijacks our RNA to multiply within our body. The cell then explodes, releasing thousands of replica viruses into the bloodstream, which then repeat the dreadful deed. They work like a stealth bomber.

To counter this, elderberries are rich in certain flavonoids, which are able to bind to the virus and block its entry into our cells.[1]

The berries are rich in vitamin C, and are able to stimulate our immune system to produce antibodies against the virus. Studies have repeatedly shown that people who have taken an elderberry preparation within 48 hours of starting a cold or flu have a reduction in their symptoms within 2 days, as compared to the normal 6 days.[2]

With some flu viruses, there is a concern that the immune system might become overstimulated, and promote a massive inflammatory reaction which can ultimately kill the victim. This is called a cytokine storm. Elderberry modulates the immune system so that it stimulates it whilst at the same time dampening an overreaction, and thereby alleviating a cytokine storm.

In addition to its antiviral properties, elderberry is also effective against pathogenic bacteria. Under laboratory conditions in Germany, elderberry was shown to be very effective against several bacteria that are responsible for pneumonia during flu-like infections, and against influenza viruses.[3]

Elderberries are like gold growing on trees. In fact, they are better than gold, because gold cannot help you against a virus, whereas elderberries can. During the 2020 Covid-19 pandemic, when my stocks of elderberries quickly ran out, you could not buy elderberries for money, but you could with love, if your supplier liked you enough to send you the last of their supplies.

But for you, dear reader, there are few nicer tasks than to go out into the gentle late summer afternoons, and collect a basketful of elderberries, absolutely free, thanks to nature's bounty. In times gone by, the berries were used to produce a rather excellent fake port! So, they can taste pretty good. Bring them home to brew into a spicy cordial, to be stored away for the cold winter days.

## ELDERBERRY GLYCERITE

**Alcohol and vinegar are not appropriate for children, but I find that the sweet softness of glycerine appeals to young palates. Elderberry glycerite is one of my favourite immune tonics for children.**

**Using dried elderberries:** Place a cup of dried elderberries in a saucepan and then add a cup of boiling water. Leave overnight with the lid on to absorb the moisture. You may need to add a little more water, until you have a consistency which enables you to blend finely with an immersion blender into a rich purple pulp. Using a sieve and a piece of muslin, strain the fluid from the berry pulp, and retain the juice. Pour the juice into a jug and add the same amount of vegetable glycerite as there is fluid. Shake and label carefully.

**Using fresh elderberries:** If you are using fresh berries, then add half a cup of boiling water to two cups of berries, bring to the boil, then switch off the heat. When cool, you can either use a potato crusher or an immersion blender to release the juice from the berries. Strain through muslin into a jug and then measure the juice, and add to this the same amount of vegetable glycerine. Mix thoroughly and bottle.

**Tip:** It is always useful to label all ingredients, and the date. If you have wild-harvested, it can be helpful to make a note of where you found your herbs, so that you can collect next year.

**Dosage:** Adults can take 1 teaspoon 4 times a day if they have a virus, or just 1 tablespoon daily as a preventative. Children under 10 years old can take 1 teaspoon twice a day if they have a virus, or 1 teaspoon daily as a preventative.

## ELDERBERRY ROB

This is a favourite of mine, and brewing it is a wonderful way to stir away a chilly evening – filling your home with the aroma of berries and spices. Elderberry rob was noted as a remedy in the ancient manuscripts which I had the privilege to read some years ago. So, this is as old as time itself. In those days, they would have used honey, so if you want to substitute the sugar for honey, that will be a more expensive but much better product. However, it might ferment more easily.

Once you have got your berry hoard back home to your kitchen, start to boil a pot of water, and with a fork, pull the berries off the stalks into the water. Throw away the green stalks. Fill your pot with a good amount of berries because you want a rich syrup.

Now gently simmer until the berries soften, then crush them with a potato masher. Switch off the heat and allow the water to extract from the berries. Once cooled, strain off the pulp, but keep the precious ruby-red liquid.

Now reheat, and stir in as much sugar as you can until it will no longer dissolve, roughly the same weight as the berries. This is your preservative. Then, add a good amount of cinnamon, crushed cloves, lemon peel, quite a lot of fresh ginger, and a few star anise pods.

Cover the pot, switch off the heat and leave overnight to cool, then strain off the spices and bottle.

**Dosage:** This delicious elixir can be taken every night over winter as an antiviral hot toddy. Because it is so sweet, it is best taken in a mug of boiling water with about 2 tablespoons of the rob in a mug.

# Turmeric (*Curcuma longa*)

These days it is quite easy to find fresh turmeric in supermarkets and greengrocers. This warming golden spice is a very useful root because it both inhibits the entry of the virus into our lung cells, as well as the replication of the virus within. But it does something else which is very important: it inhibits fibrosis (scarring). With a Covid-19 or SARS chest infection, the lung tissue becomes inflamed; this is why breathing is so laboured and difficult. But then, the inflammation hardens into scar tissue, and this is one of the aspects of the illness which leaves long-term damage. This is therefore crucial to avoid, and one of the best herbs for it is turmeric.[4][5]

## TURMERIC HOT TODDY

This is a delicious, cosy bedtime drink. In winter, when our resources are at their lowest ebb, you will find this deeply warming and comforting. Ginger and turmeric have strong antiviral properties, and warm our cold bodies during the last soggy days of winter. Both roots are strongly anti-inflammatory, which is great for aching joints, especially for those who feel creaky during cold, wet months.

Finely grate a small knob each of fresh turmeric (if you can't get fresh turmeric, then use ½ teaspoon of dried powder) and ginger root.

Add to this a cup of warm coconut, oat, almond or dairy milk, and add a grind of black pepper to release the active constituents of the turmeric.

Keep the milk on a low heat for a few minutes, with a lid covering it, to allow the antiviral constituents to infuse into your milk. It will then turn a lovely golden colour.

Now strain the milk, add a dash of cinnamon powder, and a little stevia or honey for sweetness.

Enjoy snuggled in bed!

## REFRESHING ANTIVIRAL TEA

This herbal tea is stuffed with powerful antiviral kitchen herbs and spices. You will find it an invigorating infusion to begin your day with.

½ tsp cinnamon powder

a sprig of fresh rosemary

1 clove, crushed

1 star anise

6 slices of ginger

½ tsp grated turmeric

a grind of black pepper

1 slice of lemon

Put all your aromatics in a teapot, or in a mug covered with a saucer (this keeps the all-important essential oils in the water) and pour over a cup of boiling water. When cool enough, enjoy.

# Olive leaf (*Olea europaea*)

If you visit the Mediterranean, try to harvest (with permission) some olive leaves, for they powerfully protect us from virus invasion by preventing the entry of the virus into our cells.[6] It is thought that they do this by changing the properties of the viral wall, so that the virus cannot attach to or enter our cells. Isn't that fantastic? Olive leaves can be taken as a tea, or you can make a tincture from them.

# Echinacea

For most of my career, I understood that it is the root but not the tops of echinacea which have the immune-boosting effects. But now the consensus is that echinacea preparations can have either immune-stimulating or immune-modulating effects depending on which part of the plant is used. This is important because an overstimulated immune system may initiate a dangerously high inflammatory response – a cytokine storm. It seems that echinacea has clever mechanisms which alleviate this action, and have in fact been shown to dampen down a cytokine storm.

Like all herbs, echinacea is made up of a complex chemical composition which differs between the roots, leaves and flowers. The leaves and flowers have the highest content of polysaccharides and lipoproteins, and these are responsible for the immune-stimulating effects. Not only do those gorgeous purple flowers stimulate our immune system to fight the bugs, but they act like nightclub bouncers, directly blocking and preventing the entry of the viruses into our cells.

The roots have quite a different action. They are rich in alkamides, which also have antiviral actions, but critically, they show anti-inflammatory actions and modulate the immune system. So instead of the immune system being overstimulated, the roots calm the excessive inflammatory response which a viral attack can sometimes provoke.

The alkamides also have another interesting action – their effect on cannabinoid receptors (CB1 and CB2). By docking into CB1 receptors, these natural plant chemicals balance the immune system so that there is an enhanced immune response but without the dangerous cytokine storm. To my surprise, I discovered that echinacea is used for GAD (Generalized Anxiety Disorder).[7] When the alkamides dock into CB2 receptors, the neurotransmitter anandamide (called the bliss chemical) is increased in our brain, which significantly reduces anxiety.

Of course, when we are anxious a lot, the raised cortisol levels suppress and skew our immune system away from the antiviral action, toward a more pro-inflammatory, autoimmune response, making us less resistant to viruses.

The best echinacea medicine of all is to use herb and root together. In this way, you get a well-rounded immune support, as well as the calming effects of the anandamide on our minds. By calming our adrenal output, the immune response is rebalanced. One study illustrated this beautifully by showing the aerial parts of echinacea to be extremely effective against viruses (including coronaviruses), but most effective before the virus enters the cells. Echinacea was able to partially or completely reverse the cytokine storm, and it was even effective against the pneumonia bacteria that often follow the viral infection, again reversing the inflammatory reaction and disabling the bacteria itself.[8]

I find *Echinacea purpurea* easy to grow, but I do struggle with *Echinacea angustifolia*. There are plenty of studies to show that *Echinacea purpurea* is a very effective immune tonic, and so for your purposes, it is perfectly fine to use. Personally, I hate digging up roots, so I tend to buy my echinacea root. The flowers are gorgeous, and I have to apologize profusely as I pick them, because it breaks my heart to do so. However, I do allow half the flowers to do as they wish, and consider it a fair compromise.

With the flowering tops and root together, you have a really fantastic echinacea complex. Use the fresh herb, because the antiviral properties have been found to be 10 times higher than dried.

I have chosen to give you a water- and fat-soluble recipe because the active constituents are lipophilic and hydrophilic, and it is fine to use if you don't drink alcohol.

If you don't mind alcohol, you can simply put your herb into gin or vodka, which will extract both the water and fat-soluble constituents.

## ECHINACEA GLYCERITE

50g (1¾oz) dried echinacea root
100g (3½oz) fresh echinacea flowers
    and leaves, chopped
300ml (10½fl oz) vegetable glycerine

🌿 Place the root and flowers in a glass Kilner jar and pour over 200ml (7fl oz) of boiling water. Allow to cool.

🌿 Add the vegetable glycerine. Shake it about until the water and glycerine are well mixed together, and seal. Now leave in a sunny spot for 2 weeks, then strain.

🌿 **Dosage:** You can take 1 tablespoon of this glycerite daily as an immune tonic.

## Garlic (*Allium sativum*)

Garlic is well known to have antibacterial, antiprotozoal, antifungal and antiviral properties, and is specifically antiviral against the influenza virus, cytomegalovirus, rhinovirus, herpes simplex, viral pneumonia and rotavirus. It is cheap and readily available, but quite smelly. Below is a fabulous recipe which captures the strength of the garlic but is quite palatable. It also harnesses the antiviral and antibacterial properties of honey, which (at the time of writing) was being investigated at Cairo University for its efficacy against coronavirus.[9]

### GARLIC HONEY

You need a jar of raw (unpasteurized) runny honey, and a bulb of organic garlic.

Peel all the garlic cloves and push them under the honey in the jar.

In the first 3 days, the garlic will keep bobbing to the top, so turn the jar on its head as often as possible, trying to keep the garlic under the honey.

After this you will find that the honey becomes more fluid, as the garlic juices leach into it.

As an immune tonic, take 1 teaspoon of this garlic honey morning and evening. It is quite strong-tasting but pleasant.

**CAUTION:** Be careful of taking this remedy if you are on blood thinners as garlic exacerbates the effect.

## Blackberries (*Rubus fruticosus*)

Do go out and pick basketfuls of blackberries because research shows blackberries to be an amazing superfood. The berries can be stored in your freezer and added to smoothies, turned into ice cream or enjoyed simply as a fruit.

These beloved berries of the hedgerows are highly antioxidant and anti-inflammatory, rich in vitamin C, iron and ellagic acid, which has anti-cancer effects. The blackberry tannins make them helpful in counteracting oral infections, diarrhoea and sore throats, and they have been shown to reduce gastric ulcers caused by the *Helicobacter pylori* bacteria by 88 per cent.[10]

In 2017, a young Irish student, Simon Meehan, won the BT Young Scientist of the year for discovering that the blackberry plant is a natural antibiotic against the superbug MRSA (methicillin-resistant *Staphylococcus aureus*).

Scientists have also demonstrated that blackberries have antiviral effects against the herpes simplex virus.[11] An extract of blackberry reduces the viral replication of the HSV by over 99 per cent. If you have a fresh blackberry to hand, try crushing it and applying the juice to the affected area. It would be absolutely fine to collect a bagful in the late summer and keep them frozen until such time as you may need to use them.

Plants endlessly amaze me. You have no doubt noticed how cosy you feel when eating a lovely blackberry crumble. Besides the delicious comfort-food quality of the pudding, they have also been shown to reduce anxiety.

## Lemon balm (*Melissa officinalis*)

This delightful herb (aka Melissa) is very easy to grow, and has a light, refreshing taste. It also happens to be a powerful antiviral medicine which is being considered by scientists as a future medicine against influenza viruses. The herb has another wonderful benefit, in that it calms anxiety. As I write, we are in the throes of the coronavirus pandemic, and people are very worried and upset about becoming ill. Melissa seems to work best when it comes into direct contact with the virus, and since one of the major symptoms of the coronavirus is that it affects the digestive system, with symptoms such as lack of appetite, diarrhoea, vomiting and abdominal pain, taking this herb as a tea would be potentially very beneficial. Another benefit to Melissa is its calming effects on the nervous system, which in this current climate of high anxiety makes it a herb to appreciate.

Lemon balm does not dry well, in that it seems to lose the fresh lemony essential oils which carry the antiviral constituents. That being the case, you can make a strong infusion and freeze it into ice cubes, which can later be either sucked, or popped into a cup of warm water and sipped as a herbal tea.

# SORE THROAT
The common cold often starts with a sore throat, and it is good to nip that in the bud, if we know how.

## Sage (*Salvia officinalis*)
Common old sage, which grows in your garden, is a marvel growing right under your nose. Modern science has found that this herb reduces blood sugar by increasing our sensitivity to insulin; reduces cholesterol; has anti-cancer properties; helps to slow the progression of Alzheimer's disease by improving brain cognition; eases menopausal hot flushes, and has a host of other benefits. However, in cottage medicine, it is best known as a remedy for sore throats.

The leaf has a strong and pungent fragrance, which tells us that it is full of volatile oils. These oils are powerfully antibacterial and antiviral. The leaves also have tannins, which tighten swollen and engorged mucous membrane tissues, thereby reducing inflammation. Tannins can kill bacteria by changing their protein structure in a similar way to cooking. But there is more that the humble sage gives us: the plant is even able to reduce the pain sensation of sore throats – this action being called antinociceptive. So, when you pick some leaves, do give it a stroke of appreciation, for it is a generous and powerful ally.

## SAGE AND CINNAMON TEA

This is a quick and very effective little kitchen remedy for sore throats.

1 tsp fresh sage leaves, or ½ tsp
   dried leaves
½ tsp cinnamon powder

Put the sage and cinnamon in a teapot, pour over a cup of boiling water and quickly cover. When cool enough, strain and gargle.

This is important: A sore throat is covered with bacteria or viruses, and you don't really want to swallow them. So, for the first mouthful, you gargle and spit it out. Thereafter, you gargle and swallow so that the healing herbal liquid covers the throat and also enters the bloodstream.

**CAUTION:** Do not use sage if you are pregnant.

## LOVELY LEMON BALM TEA

In the height of summer, collect your lemon balm and chop it roughly, so that you have 1 cup of freshly chopped lemon balm leaves.

You might like to add fresh ginger to support lemon balm's antiviral action on the gut lining. If so, finely chop 2 tablespoons of fresh ginger.

Place in a large teapot and add 2 cups of boiling water, then quickly replace the lid. After an hour, strain this tea, then pour into an ice-cube tray to freeze for later, or add a little honey to taste and chill to serve as a delicious iced tea for summer afternoons.

# Rowan berries
## (*Sorbus aucuparia*)

For generations the rowan tree has been associated with witches and the faery folk. Some still say that the faeries live in the tree, or that it marks an entrance into their underworld. It has long been used as a tree of protection against witches, and country folk used to tie rowan twigs into a cross with a red thread and nail the talisman above doorways and in barns. They even wove it into their horses' manes to prevent them from being hag-ridden during the night.

On a more therapeutic level, rowan berry syrup has a tradition of being used to relieve sore throats. It is rich in antioxidants, which help to reduce inflammation in the throat and respiratory tract, and a singers' syrup made from the berries was valued for its effects on soothing hoarseness of the throat, presumably producing silky sounds from the owner of the vocal cords. It is so packed with vitamin C that it was also used to treat scurvy.

The berries contain parasorbic acid, which is poisonous to the kidneys, but upon heating, parasorbic acid changes to harmless sorbic acid – therefore it is very important that the berries are cooked for quite a while (as you do when making jam). The seeds are also toxic, so they should be carefully strained out. After that, you will have a delicious jelly with a wild tart flavour which matches splendidly with pork sausages or strong cheddar. Don't be afraid to use this berry. I have made Rowan jelly year after year, and each autumn we eagerly look forward to our rowan berry jelly with farm sausages. These days we are all scaredy-cats. Let's go feral instead!

## ROWAN BERRY AND CLOVE SYRUP
**Collect the plump red/orange berries at the end of summer.**

Strip the berries from the twigs and rinse them in cold water. Now place 2 cups of berries in a saucepan and add enough water to cover the berries, then bring to the boil. Turn down the heat and simmer, adding 1 tablespoon of cloves at this stage (cloves are strongly antimicrobial but they also have a slight numbing effect which is very comforting when you have a raw sore throat), and place the lid on until the berries turn soft. You can even squash them with a potato masher. Make sure that the berries are completely cooked through – you will see little brown seeds floating about at this stage.

Strain the pulp through a fine sieve making sure that all the seeds and cloves have been collected, and discard them. Return the pulp to the pan, and perhaps add a little more water, then keep adding sugar to the liquid until it will no longer dissolve. Pour into bottles and seal.

Add 20ml (1 tablespoon plus 1 teaspoon) of syrup to a glass of warm water, and sip to soothe your sore throat. You can make this more effective if you add the 20ml to a cup of sage and cinnamon tea (see page 25).

*Rowan berry syrup has a tradition of being used to relieve sore throats. It is rich in antioxidants, which help to reduce inflammation in the throat and respiratory tract.*

## ROWAN BERRY JELLY

**This is really a culinary jelly, but it is so delightful that I don't want you to miss out on the recipe.**

Collect nice red berries, pull them off the stalks, and rinse.

Hopefully you can locate some wild apples. I have to compete for apples with the cows who break out of their field to enjoy the apples off a certain tree down my lane. If you can't find wild apples, perhaps scrump some from your neighbour's tree, and as a last resort, buy some.

Roughly chop the apples, skin, pips and all. Put the berries and apples in a saucepan with a little water and bring to the boil. I haven't given quantities, because it is a matter of choice how much you make. Add jam sugar and keep boiling until the fruit collapses. To test if your jelly will set, drop a small amount onto a cold plate and wait a minute or two, then gently push the blob with your finger. If it is thick and wrinkles, then it will set. If the blob does not form wrinkles, keep boiling for a few more minutes, then test again.

In the meantime, carefully wash your glass jars and place in an oven at 140ºC (275ºF) to sterilize.

When the jelly is ready, take the jars out of the oven. At this stage, I usually add a few sage leaves or a large bay leaf to each jar, then pour the hot fruit mixture through a fine sieve, into a heatproof glass or ceramic jug, and from there, directly into the jars. The leaf will sizzle and sputter dramatically, so do stand back. One the drama has ceased, seal the jar with the lid.

# SINUS AND CHEST INFECTIONS

## Horseradish (*Armoracia rusticana*)

Once you have horseradish in your garden, you will always have it. The taproot penetrates very deeply into the soil, and however far you dig, a tiny bit always remains to grow again. Which is just as well, because it is a most underrated herb. Traditionally, horseradish has been used to treat bladder and chest infections.

Grate the root, and the pungent vapours assault your nose with such a robust force that you are left in no doubt as to the power of this root to kill. Within the tissues of the root is sinigrin, which is cleverly separated from the enzyme myrosinase within the cells. When the two are combined, they instantly form a potent mustard vapour which is extremely repellent to browsing herbivores. However, as medicine makers, we actively seek to harvest these natural chemicals for our own benefit. This is why we carefully grate the root, because that breaks down the cell structure, allowing sinigrin and the enzyme to combine into a medicine which boosts the immune system, kills viruses, bacteria and fungi, and also fights against cancer.[12]

The pungent mustard oils slightly irritate the mucous membranes of the sinuses and lungs, causing the cells to secrete a thin fluid which dislodges thick sticky phlegm, promoting the coughing up or blowing out of the infected mucus. At the same time, as we eat the root, the mustard oils are absorbed into our bloodstream and then breathed off via our lungs, killing the offending bacteria and virus.

## HORSERADISH VINEGAR

**If you don't have horseradish in your garden, at Christmas time, you can often purchase some from a greengrocer.**

Grate the root, taking care to keep your eyes away from the rising fumes. Quickly place in a glass jar.

In the meantime, gently heat 500ml (2 cups) of good-quality apple cider vinegar. Just warm and do not bring to the boil because the vinegar is a living product, and we want to preserve the healing qualities of all our ingredients.

Now pour the warm vinegar over the grated root, and quickly seal the jar to avoid your eyeballs being scorched. Macerate (steep) for 3 days before straining into a glass bottle.

Horseradish vinegar can be taken with honey and a little water, or by simply adding to hot water to sip as a tea, which is much more pleasant than you might imagine. Do not drink this without diluting.

**Dosage:** For a nasty cough with thick sticky mucus, or for a sinus infection, the dose is 1 tablespoon 4 times a day for adults.

## DRAGON'S BLOOD CHEST CLEANSER

It's red and fiery, and immensely effective against chesty viral infections. This little concoction stimulates the immune system to eliminate the virus or bacteria, whilst the herbs directly disable the bugs. It also loosens the thick sticky phlegm which forms a comfortable home for bacteria, thus cleansing your lungs and sinus cavities, leaving you feeling much clearer and able to breathe more easily. For those of you with weak chests, this recipe can be taken throughout the winter to protect your lungs.

Simply combine half horseradish vinegar with half elderberry rob or elderberry glycerine for a pleasantly bracing but impressively powerful medicine.

If you are ill, then take 1 teaspoon 4 times a day. As a cold and flu preventative, take 1 tablespoon daily.

## HORSERADISH TEA

Go back to your horseradish vinegar. Add 1 teaspoon of horseradish vinegar to a cup of boiling water, and while you are waiting for the water to cool down, softly cup your hands around the mug to capture the steam and inhale (without scorching your eyeballs), then drink it as hot as you can without burning your mouth. You will find this causes your nasal passages to discharge thick sticky mucus.

If you happen to have dried elderflowers in the house, add a teaspoon or two to your mug, as these will most marvellously help to bring down the inflammation of your mucous membranes, and this in itself will relieve the pain and congestion.

Drink this tea 4 to 6 times a day whilst you have sinus pain.

## Elecampane (*Inula helenium*)

Elecampane is my number one herb for chest infections. In ancient times, this plant was known as elfwort, and it was the antidote to elfshot. Wort is derived from the Anglo-Saxon word *wyrt*, meaning "herb". So, this was a herb to cure illness caused by elves. In those days, elves were unseen but very real and powerful creatures, which, if displeased, might shoot invisible arrows into their victim. Elfshot would cause illness or possibly even death, unless those attending the victim knew the right herbs (and incantations) to use to avert such an event. The elf arrows were invisible, but clearly felt as a sudden sharp pain in the side of the chest. The puncture wound caused the life force to pour out, but the victim's body would try to compensate by generating a fierce heat (we call this a fever), which ran up along the spine to the head like molten lava.

Today, we call the above illness pleurisy, and possibly pneumonia, and the plant is known as elecampane. It has powerful antibacterial and expectorant properties, and I have used it many times to cure chest infections. I find it particularly useful for those who have had a chest infection for months, and are severely weakened by the illness. This plant has power.

Inula is my final harvest of the season. The plant is stately, and I carefully lift it from the soil and snip off the thick, finger-like roots. I then replace the plant in its bed, and cover it with a thick mulch of manure in thanks for the treasure which it has given me.

The snipped roots are scrubbed thoroughly, then, with a very sharp knife, I slice the root length-ways. These curls of roots, which look like witches' fingernails, are left to dry on a cloth in my apothecary. Once dried, I turn them into a medicine in the form of syrup, tincture or elecampane balls. The dried elecampane shavings can be powdered in a coffee grinder for the recipe opposite.

## ELFWORT BALLS

1 tsp elecampane powder
1 tsp marshmallow root, or
    slippery elm bark powder
1 tsp liquorice root powder

In a small bowl, mix all the powders together so that they are evenly distributed. Now, sprinkle in a few drops of warm water, and mix. Keep doing this until you have a stiff paste. Then knead and roll the paste into small hazelnut-sized balls, and leave to dry on a plate.

The elecampane will help to kill the infection and expectorate the phlegm. The marshmallow or slippery elm and the liquorice will soothe a raw, sore bronchial lining, also helping to expectorate the thick sticky mucus.

Once dry, these handy little balls are very convenient to keep in a small sweet tin in your car, desk drawer or handbag, and sucked, with great effect, if you have a chest infection.

## Onions (*Allium cepa*)

The use of onions as a medicine goes back as far as Dioscorides in the 1st century, and even further, to ancient Mesopotamia. They are well documented as being effective against stomach cancer, diabetes and menopausal osteoporosis, or even soothing to piles when made into an ointment with hemp, hot sesame oil and turmeric. (I haven't dared to try this recipe on any haemorrhoid sufferers.)

Many of my older patients have told me how they were effectively treated for childhood whooping cough, bronchitis or asthma with a simple remedy called onion syrup. This is the recipe which I often suggest to people who call me when I am away from my apothecary for a few days, and unable to send herbs. It is quick to make and quick to help.

## ONION SYRUP FOR A CHILD'S COUGH

🌿 Cut one organic strong white onion into thick slices. Do not break the slices up into rings, but layer the onion slices with sugar in a glass or ceramic bowl. It doesn't matter if you use dark brown or white sugar, just sprinkle thick layers of sugar between the onion slices, cover with a plate, and leave to extract overnight.

🌿 In the morning you will find a bowl with onion syrup. Discard the onion rings and keep the syrup in the refrigerator. A child can have 1 teaspoon every 2 hours if the cough is severe, or 3 times a day if the cough is mild, or nearly finished.

# Wild garlic (*Allium ursinum*)

I think that all across the land, we eagerly await the coming of wild garlic (aka ramsons) in the spring. The hills are festooned with the gorgeous glossy leaves, and later the beautiful white lily-like flowers. Almost everyone I know has their springtime ritual of wild garlic soup or pesto. Here are my recipes for both, for they both marvellously boost the constitution! Wild garlic has all the medical properties of kitchen garlic and is possibly even more antiviral, antibacterial, antifungal and antiparasitic. It is excellent to eat if you have a chest or sinus infection. This is a really good example of letting food be your medicine.

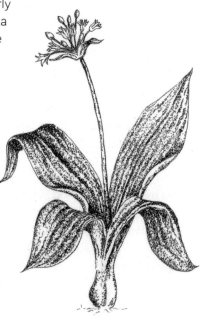

## FOREST-FLOOR PESTO

generous handful of wild garlic leaves
(be careful to pick away from the
path so that you do not collect
leaves upon which dogs have
lifted their legs)
plenty of olive oil
walnuts, crushed
Parmesan cheese, finely grated

🌿 Blend the wild garlic leaves with the olive oil until you have a fairly rough consistency. Add the crushed nuts and whizz again. Then add the grated cheese, and give a final whizz.

🌿 Eat immediately or freeze. We found this makes a really novel gift when visiting friends or family.

## WILD GARLIC SOUP

This soup is ultra-comforting if you are feeling fragile and in need of a hearty soup, so it is a good idea to make plenty and freeze some.

🌿 Make a good chicken or mushroom stock as described earlier (see page 13). Make sure that the chicken has cooked long and slow so that you have a lovely thick stock.

🌿 Now add some peeled potatoes, and allow to cook until soft, and perhaps some shiitake mushrooms, then add as many handfuls of wild garlic leaves as you can get into the soup. They will quickly wilt, and then you can run a hand blender through the soup so that it becomes silky smooth. You might like to add a whirl of cream to enrich this deliciously healing soup.

# Jack-by-the-hedge (*Alliaria petiolata*)

Garlic mustard, aka Jack-by-the-hedge, is a herb which you are very likely to find if you are of the wandering kind who packs a thermos flask and a few sandwiches to sustain a long walk in the early months of spring. This common little plant is generally to be found tucked away under a hedge, looking as inconspicuous as possible, avoiding attention and devouring. Once discovered, the wayfarer looks eagerly for Jack-by-the-hedge thereafter. The tender green leaves taste fairly strongly of garlic with enough heat to justify the mustard part of the name. They are delicious when added to your picnic sandwich, snipped into cream cheese on an oat biscuit or tossed into a herby omelette, and are very nice with sour cream and smoked salmon.

The herb was valued in the past to treat sore throats, pneumonia and coughs. Indeed, a chest infection craves garlic, which is powerfully antibiotic and antiviral. This often-unacknowledged wayside herb kills the invading bacteria, dislodges the mucus in which the bacteria proliferate, promotes the expectoration of the infected mucus and dilates the bronchi.

In the case of a cold, this punchy snack will help to kill the bacteria in your lungs or sinuses.

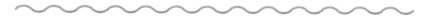

## JACK ON TOAST

Toast a slice of rye bread, and rub both sides with a clove of raw garlic. Mash an avocado and include in the mash plenty of finely chopped "Jack" and wild garlic if you can find some, as well as ¼ teaspoon of horseradish sauce.

Pile the mash onto the toast and enjoy. It is pungent, but you will immediately feel your respiratory passages opening and the mucus shifting.

## Thyme (*Thymus vulgaris*)

Thyme, and hyssop too, are both excellent herbs to beat off sinus and chest infections. They help to fight the bacteria and viruses, and at the same time, loosen thick sticky phlegm, so that it can more easily be expelled. Both grow easily in the garden, and can be dried or used fresh. They are probably best taken as a hot infusion because you can inhale the essential-oil-rich steam before you drink the tea.

🌿 Use 1 teaspoon of herb per cup of boiling water. As soon as you pour the boiling water over the herb, the little glands holding essential oils within the leaf will rupture, releasing the healing vapours. These vaporized volatile oils can be captured either by placing a towel over your head like a tent, and breathing in the fragrant steamy air, or by cupping your hands around the mug and placing your mouth and nose over your cupped hands to inhale the steam. Once the brew is cool enough, you can drink it. Do this 3–5 times a day.

🌿 **CAUTION:** Avoid hyssop if you have ever had a seizure, as it may trigger another. Avoid thyme if you have an oestrogen-driven cancer. Avoid both if you are pregnant.

~~~~~~~~~~

### KITCHEN–CUPBOARD REMEDY FOR SINUS AND CHEST INFECTIONS

1 tsp dried thyme (antibacterial)

2.5cm (1in) of fresh ginger, grated (anti-bacterial and antiviral, warms the chest)

½ tsp horseradish sauce, or 1 tsp horseradish vinegar (decongests the passages)

1cm (½in) fresh turmeric, grated, or ½ tsp dried (anti-inflammatory)

if you have marshmallow leaves or liquorice root, add 1 teaspoon of each (soothes raw airways)

🌿 Place this all in a teapot, and add 2 cups of boiling water. Steep for 10 minutes, then sip. You can add honey (immune-boosting and soothing) and lemon (antiviral) to taste.

# EAR INFECTIONS

You can't mess around with ear infections. See a doctor as soon as possible, but these two remedies will give the patient some relief until the antibiotics kick in.

~~~~~~~~~~~~~~~~~~~~~~~~~~~~~~

## FOR CHILDREN: ROASTED ONION

Roast a strong white organic onion. When warmed through, cut in half and allow to cool so that it will not scald the child's skin.

Now cover with a clean cloth such as folded muslin, and place the warm onion on a towel which covers a pillow, and then let the child lie with their ear over the onion, so that the warm antibiotic steam can begin the disinfecting process.

You will find that the warmth is greatly comforting for the child, and it is at least something that you can do overnight before you get to your doctor.

~~~~~~~~~~~~~~~~~~~~~~~~~~~~~~

## FOR ADULTS: EUCALYPTUS

As a first aid, I often recommend adults rub a drop of eucalyptus essential oil behind the ear. If you run your finger from behind the earlobe and down the throat/neck, you will find a natural channel.

Running your eucalyptus-anointed finger gently but firmly in downward strokes, you will help to move the congested mucus in the Eustachian tube. The oil will diffuse into the tissues and help to kill the bacteria and viruses within the ear canals.

# SWOLLEN GLANDS

## Goosegrass (*Galium aparine*)

During a viral infection, the glands in the neck often swell up painfully. The glands lining our intestines can also swell: we are unable to feel the knobs, but will feel nauseous and put off our food. A safe and effective herb to use in this case is *Galium aparine*, known as goosegrass, clivers or sticky willy. It is a very common herb, but harvest it when you see it, because once it has seeded, it will disappear.

It used to be said that if you want to be lean and lank (like the herb), drink clivers, and indeed, it is a lymphatic decongestant and diuretic, so it helps to shift the toxins held in our cellulite. But we are talking about glands now, and this is one of my favourite herbs to use with almost any glandular condition such as tonsillitis, glandular fever or breast lumps. For swollen and tender glands, simply pick a handful of the stringy herb. Roll it into a ball and stuff it into a glass of water. Leave overnight and drink during the day. I would recommend drinking at least three of these glasses if you have swollen glands.

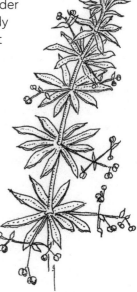

To preserve this herb, extracting it in apple cider vinegar would be a good option. Pull the weedy herb out of the hedge and allow it to dry out for a day or two because it is very watery (like cucumber) and this can dilute the preserving action of the vinegar. Then roughly chop up and stuff a Kilner jar with the herb, and pour warmed apple cider vinegar over the plant matter.

Seal the jar and leave in a sunny place for at least two weeks. Keep an eye on your medicine to make sure that it doesn't turn mouldy. Then, press out and filter through muslin, and bottle. The dose would be 1 tablespoon four times a day to cleanse enlarged and painful glands.

# TAKE A TIP FROM FOUR THIEVES

The 17th century was a terrible time when the Black Death killed almost half the population of Eurasia. Whilst everyone suffered during this awful time, four thieves prospered.

Seemingly immune from the disease, they entered the homes of the dead and dying and robbed them of their valuable goods. Eventually they were caught and sentenced to be burned at the stake. However, they were offered the quicker and less painful death by hanging if they revealed their secret recipe. It was a herbal vinegar, which they rubbed "on their hands, ears and temples from time to time when approaching a plague victim".

This preparation became known as *Acetum Anti-Septicum vulgo des Quatre Voleurs* (Vinegar of the Four Thieves), and was made up of wormwood, rosemary, sage, mint, rue, lavender, garlic, cinnamon, cloves, nutmeg and calamus, macerated in vinegar for 12 days and then strained. After that, camphor dissolved in spirit was added. Now the thieves were ready to help themselves to the belongings of others with impunity, as long as they repeatedly washed their hands, nose and mouth with the vinegar.

The vinegar preparation was used for at least 200 years after that date, particularly by those who had to "haunt infected places and attend those who were at risk of death, such as churches, prisons, ships, and places of amusement". In 1819, the medical pharmacopoeia of Edinburgh dropped the garlic and called it "Acetum Aromaticum". Eventually the preparation was made with essential oils of juniper, lavender, mint, rosemary, citrus and clove.

If we are still in a pandemic at the time of you reading this book, then you might find this vinegar helpful to carry in your car or handbag. But even during a normal cold and flu season, it will help to mitigate the effects of other people's bugs left on trolley handles, etc.

## FOUR THIEVES VINEGAR

**Use the following essential oils:**

10 drops of rosemary
10 drops of tea tree
10 drops of Scots pine
8 drops of lavender
5 drops of lemon peel
3 drops of clove
3 drops of peppermint
2 drops of cinnamon

Add this blend of essential oils to 100ml (3½fl oz) of vinegar, and carefully pour into a glass bottle. Shake before applying to your hands.

**CAUTION:** Do not use if pregnant, and if you are prone to epilepsy leave out the rosemary.

## PROTECTING YOURSELF WHEN OUT AND ABOUT

In the not-so-long-ago days, people would walk around with a piece of garlic tied around their neck. This is very effective at cleansing your personal air space, but probably not very socially attractive – although that might be desirable too!

Another option is to make yourself an antiviral/antibacterial spritz, which you can keep in your handbag or car to spray your hands, steering wheel, shopping trolley, etc.

## PINE, FIR AND EUCALYPTUS ESSENTIAL OILS

These are great essential oils which help to open up the airways. They also help to fight bacteria lurking in the passages of your sinuses, and protect you against other people's germs. They smell nice and fresh too.

As a first defence against a sinus infection, add a drop of each to a tissue and sniff deeply, or if you are wearing dark colours, add the drops to your collar, so that the essential oils vaporize around you all day. Personally, I just apply them neat under my nostrils where they float straight up the nose and clear the passages.

## HERBAL CHEST RUB

Essential oils are excellent for defending yourself against respiratory tract infections because they vaporize straight into the respiratory tract where the bacteria and viruses hang out. If you are going out, into public spaces like trains or airports, you might like to make this little blend of essential oils. If you are wearing a mask, then add a drop onto your mask.

1 drop each of eucalyptus, pine, thyme, tea tree and lavender (personally, I would make a little bottle of equal quantities of each – it's simpler).

Add 5 drops of this blend to 1 teaspoon of kitchen olive oil and anoint your chest – front and back. Or add 3 drops of this blend to a bowl of hot water, cover your head with a towel and breathe gently for a few minutes.

You can also vaporize these oils in a diffuser when you get home. If you don't have a diffuser, don't worry. Add a few drops onto a slightly damp cloth and hang over a radiator. That will help to kill the bugs in the air and also disinfect your airways.

# MUSTARD BATH

A mustard bath is a marvellous Victorian recipe, which is ultra-comforting when you are suffering from those aches and chills caused by winter viruses. If you don't have a bath, you can make a foot bath, and the beneficial magnesium salts will be absorbed through the soles of your feet, while the essential oils will evaporate up into your nasal and lung passages.

The bath salts are made from magnesium-rich Epsom salts, which open the pores in our skin and allow the toxins to perspire out. The magnesium is also an effective muscle relaxer, soothing pain and tension.

Place a double handful of Epsom salts in a glass or ceramic bowl, then mix in 2 heaped tablespoons of sieved English mustard powder. Now that you have your base, add the blend listed below, or other essential oils of your choice. Once the oils have been added to the salts, stir in vigorously with a spoon, and then seal in a glass jar.

Now run your bath, and just as you get into the warm water, add all your fragrant salts, and surrender to the healing power of plants. Use this bath when you feel that bone-aching chilly feeling, with a stuffed-up nose. It is a firm favourite amongst my patients.

## MUSTARD BATH ESSENTIAL-OIL BLEND

20 drops of eucalyptus essential oil (leave out this ingredient if pregnant or prone to epilepsy)

20 drops of lavender essential oil

20 drops of pine essential oil

10 drops of peppermint essential oil

# A SELF-NURTURING RITUAL
# FOR WHEN YOU ARE FEELING AWFUL

If it is one of those dark, bone-piercingly cold, wet winter days, and you feel run-down and exhausted, hopefully you would have made some of the recipes above to call upon.

Warm yourself a bowl of nourishing broth, and either switch on your electric blanket or slip a cosy hot-water bottle into your bed. Enjoy the richly nourishing soup and then run a bath. Once the tub is full, add your mustard bath salts and sink in for at least 20 minutes, listening to some gentle music to calm your brainwaves. I find solfeggio music, and also Indian chanting yoga music, very peaceful. It calms my brainwaves and gives a sense of peacefulness which can be quite rare these days for most people.

If you don't bathe, then warm yourself under a hot shower. Wrap up and then place a handful of mustard bath salts into a wide bowl so that you can soak your feet in this while you enjoy a bowl of nourishing soup.

When you are ready for bed, pour some boiling water over your elderberry rob, or make a cosy turmeric hot toddy – use your instinct to choose which. Then get into bed with your warming, healing drink, a gentle book and read yourself to sleep. If you do have a virus, allow yourself to sweat it out all night.

Viruses cannot survive elevated body temperatures, which is why we develop fevers. This is our body's clever response to the virus. So, allow yourself to sweat all night, and in the morning, have a shower or bath, and change your sheets. You will need to have a gentle day to recover, so this is a day of more nourishing soups and herbal teas. If you really have to work, perhaps you could work from home, with shorter hours.

## POST-VIRAL FATIGUE

This is a condition that really requires professional help. Some people who contracted the coronavirus are suffering from long Covid, which seems to be a type of post-viral fatigue, along with a list of other symptoms, often quite varied. In such a case, as with chronic fatigue syndrome and post-viral fatigue, I really do recommend that you see a professional medical herbalist or other well-qualified health professional to help you through this. Having said that, there is a tradition that sloes, and the small green shoots from blackthorn bushes, are an excellent tonic for those who feel sluggish and exhausted following a bacterial and viral attack. Sloes are a great tonic and a cleanser of the body, so do collect your sloes in November and make yourself a nice batch of sloe gin, if only for medicinal purposes.

## NOURISHING YOUR ADRENALS

The adrenal glands should be of major consideration in our day and age. One hundred years ago, people were bored to shrieks because nothing much happened in their villages. Much the same happens in my village, where if a heron eats all the fish in the pond, we are all agog with the news! Personally, I like it that way.

But for most of us, these days, there is so much change in our everyday lives that we cannot keep up. We are expected to do so much, and we expect to achieve so much, that most people are completely overwhelmed. Beyond that, the media soaks into our subconscious words like "terror", "uncertainty" and "pandemic", which are used over and over for years, until the public feels uncertain and terrified. This leads to a vague but unremitting sense of anxiety and fear of life itself. In order to defend against the uncertainty of life, people whizz around doing more and more, burning up their inner resources, forgetting that life is to be lived and enjoyed. The work-life balance is utterly thrown out of kilter in the striving for survival in our crazy world.

In my experience, most people are quite unaware of their subconscious overwhelm until they "hit the wall" and become so exhausted and burned out that they literally cannot do another day of it.

Of course, mainstream medicine knows about the adrenal glands, and so gives some attention to burnout, but they don't seem interested in adrenal fatigue – in fact they deny that condition. Perhaps that is because beyond advising you to take a holiday, or offering antidepressants so that you feel better about feeling awful, allopathic medicine really doesn't have anything further to offer. But nature has plenty to offer. Plants can heal us, our diet can fortify us, and our lifestyles can be adjusted to healthier choices. Spending quality time with loved ones, and taking time out to be alone, brings us back home to ourselves, and returns us to an almost forgotten and more humane pace of life. Of course, simply spending time in nature is immediately and discernibly grounding, rebalancing and restorative.

In this section, I am going to give you a brief synopsis of what happens to your body as you burn out, and how you can help yourself. However, if you do think that you suffer from adrenal fatigue, I strongly recommend that you see a medical herbalist or naturopath because they will prescribe herbal medicines and nutrients specifically for your individual condition. Having said that, there is much that can and should be done from home.

*  *  *

It doesn't follow nature to separate the body into systems such as the nervous system, the digestive system and the immune system. We separate them as a matter of convenience for examination and diagnosis, but we must remember that our body systems are intimately interlaced, communicating with each other all the time. Every cell in your body is in communication with every other cell, thus what happens to one, happens to them all.

As such, when our nervous system is alerted to danger, so too is every other cell in our body. We are designed to get a fright, deal with it, and then continue on with our lives. The sympathetic nervous system is our survivor system. When we get a fright (the lioness charges at us), our brain registers an emergency, rapid signals are sent to our adrenal glands which immediately secrete adrenaline (epinephrine) and cortisol to give us the super-human strength to run or fight. We escape, get back to our cave, tell the story to our clan and everyone falls about laughing. Thus, we recover and live another day.

Or, a neighbouring clan raids your cattle. Your clan finds out, you go and duff the other clan up, and then your tribe retaliates by stealing their cattle at another time. These sorts of incidents have always occurred sporadically and we are designed to survive them.

Life isn't like that anymore. We are almost constantly on red alert with deadlines, ringing phones, emails, bills, family dramas, traffic jams, horrifically violent films, road rage, cybercrime, outraged social media posts, caged dogs in foreign countries – the list is endless, and we feel compelled to keep on top of all of this, whilst at the same time trying to provide our family with a safe and happy life. Life is hard, even in the wealthy West.

When we live in a state of almost constant fight or flight, our adrenal glands will secrete the hormones of stress – adrenaline and cortisol. Over time, cortisol skews our immune system by downregulating our ability to fight viruses, and upregulating our susceptibility to allergies and environmental sensitivities.

The adrenaline switches off our digestive enzyme secretions and freezes the peristaltic movement of our intestines. Thus, our food does not break down as it should; instead it languishes like a brick in our stomach, fermenting, producing flatulence and toxins which make us fatigued, give us headaches and clog up the liver.

Because we are tired, we may reach for the caffeine or sugar. Under normal circumstances, a cup of coffee or two is absolutely fine, but when you are burned out, it is not fine. The caffeine will only push an already exhausted system beyond its limits. In these cases, coffee gives you "energy" but it is a false friend. It stimulates you past your capacity to carry on, and when the caffeine wears off, you are even more depleted. Every day it takes a little more than it gives.

Sugar is similar. After eating something sweet, you feel fantastic, but when the blood sugar levels drop, you feel dreadful and may reach for another food fix. With the diminished digestive enzymatic secretion caused by the overstimulation of the sympathetic nervous system, the food is not digested properly, and ferments. Because the population of our inner microbiota responds to the food we eat, the fermenting food might support strains of bacteria and yeast or fungi which are not supportive to our health. Sugar feeds the yeast, and soon you have a fungal overgrowth, such as *Candida albicans*, in your digestive system. The fungus can develop root-like structures which pierce the wall of your intestines, allowing the fungus to migrate into your bloodstream, and from there to other parts of your body, causing massive health disruptions.

With the immune system suppressed by the over-secretion of cortisol, and at the same time trying to deal with the fungal invasion, it is less able to fight off viruses and bacteria. It is at this point the virus can invade the body and really take hold, leading to problems like glandular fever, or you can have a flare-up of the normally quiet viruses, resulting in shingles or a herpes episode.

You did not get ill at this point. Your state of health was already severely depleted, but you just didn't realize it. For some people it can be very dramatic, and one day they wake up to find that they literally cannot get out of bed.

The underlying cause of adrenal fatigue is nervous overstimulation, and this can become an unsustainable habit. A reconsideration of your lifestyle is absolutely crucial to recovery. Some people choose to cut down their work, work from home, downsize and simplify their lives, change their careers from the city to becoming gardeners, drop people who drain their energy, recruit other members of their family or professionals to share in the care of elderly parents, find peace in their important relationships – you have to work out what is best for you so that you bring your life back into balance.

## Common symptoms of adrenal fatigue:

- A deep fatigue which is not relieved by sleep

- Poor-quality sleep or difficulty falling asleep, or waking with a start in the night

- Waking up feeling as tired as you felt when you went to bed last night

- Brain fog, difficulty finding words, difficulty following a conversation

- Too tired to digest your food

- Muscle aches all over your body

- Weepy, a feeling of doom or dread

- Cannot face any stress or demands, possibly leading to angry outbursts (these are more signs of desperate tiredness rather than an unpleasant personality)

- Wanting to hide from the world; wanting to give it all up and run away

- Poor wound healing, poor skin condition

- Hair loss or loss of condition

- Hormonal disturbances – excessive pre-menstrual tension or hot flushes (hormone levels have crashed), loss of libido, inability to conceive

- Never catching a cold, or, paradoxically, not being able to recover from a cold or flu

- Low blood pressure, dizziness upon standing up

- Copious pale urine

These symptoms may seem vague, and even something that you can ignore and it will go away. Almost all of my chronic fatigue (chronic means long term) patients have tried to "push past" these symptoms, but to no avail. This is a generally unrecognized condition, which leaves one believing that you are malingering, but you are not.

It is a modern problem and very common. It is serious and must be attended to. I am afraid that the best way to deal with adrenal fatigue is to surrender to it. You cannot fight your way through because that is how you became ill. By ignoring your body's requests for rest, you pushed too hard for too long and now your body just cannot give you any more leeway. The sooner you change the way you live, the sooner you will feel better. But, here's the rub: you cannot go back to the way things were. You have to re-evaluate your life and find a better way. A more humane pace of life, and a way of life that is kinder. Kindness to yourself is the key.

## KIND THINGS

When I was a child, I philosophically decided that life was full of difficulties, which I rather dramatically named "nasty things", and these needed to be offset by "kind things". I hasten to add that my life was wonderful, actually, but homework, etc. fell under the category of nasty things. I started introducing to my life as many kind things as I could, which might have included walking up the mountain, tea with a friend in the garden, a nice magazine, a fragrant bath, or an early night with a good book and a mug of hot chocolate on a wintery night. Little things which tip the balance of life; an act of self-kindness.

Hopefully you, dear reader, will never hit the wall, but it is most prudent to pay attention to how you are feeling, and give your body the respect it deserves by obeying its requests. Here are some ideas of kind things, but of course, you should choose your own.

- If you need a holiday, do what you can to take one.

- Reconnect with nature. There is enough evidence to back up what we all know, and that is that we feel better when we spend time in nature. The negative ions released by trees, waterfalls and the ocean increase our serotonin and lift our mood, relieve stress, and increase blood flow to our brain, which makes us feel brighter.

- If you need a very quiet weekend, clear your diary, switch off your phone, and potter around the garden, or cook nourishing food, or sew, or make something creative – the options are endless. Tune into what you loved or yearned to do as a child, and do that.

- Think of your bathroom as a spa – perhaps have a long Epsom salt bath or a shower and then meditate on your bed, or watch a gentle film.

- Go to bed at 6pm if that is what you need – why not, anyway? You may not fall asleep, but you can gently read and rest your body and mind.

- If your brain cannot switch off from an overstimulated and agitated state, try playing soothing music. You can find these easily on YouTube; try solfeggio music, or Indian chanting music, Gregorian chanting or soft rain music – these are specifically designed to calm down overactive brainwaves. You can literally feel your brainwaves calming back into a co-ordinated state of peace.

- Switch off all screens at least 1 hour before you sleep, and choose to read gentle books. Subjects of a peaceful and kind nature will help you to fall into a peaceful, restful and restorative sleep.

# HERBS

There are a great many options for healing and restoring the adrenal system with herbal medicine, but I am not going to list all the herbs because this is a book on home herbal medicine, and most of the herbs that we use are not found in the home. Buying herbs on the internet is a risky business because you just do not know if it is adulterated or the pure herb. A professional medical herbalist will consider your individual case, and prescribe a formula of herbs specifically for you and your unique requirements. For instance, some people burn out due to emotional exhaustion, whilst others are overworked, or have been through an exceptionally demanding period of their lives. Each of these cases would require a different approach. Having said that, there are some herbs which we can easily access, which are wonderfully nourishing and should be included in any recovery regime.

# CALMING HERBS

So many people do not reside in their bodies. They live in their heads, and those heads are somewhere in their future plans, planning future goals, thinking about what needs to get done.

There is something very peaceful about coming home to the present moment. Focusing on what you are doing right now, and trusting that by looking after the present, the future takes care of itself. One thing at a time – it is a discipline. Coming back to the present time and space is like slipping a hand in a glove – it just fits. Life becomes simple, peaceful and focused.

Calming herbs such as lemon balm, vervain, valerian, passiflora and Californian poppy can help you to come back into your body. Even the ritual of collecting the herbs, drying them, and then over the next few weeks making the infusion, is time out.

## Liquorice (*Glycyrrhiza glabra*)

The number one choice for adrenal fatigue is liquorice. Not the bags of sweets, I'm afraid, for they are mainly sugar and aniseed flavouring, but pure liquorice extract, which can easily be purchased in town or on the internet. You may find that for a time, you absolutely crave liquorice, even if you don't normally like it. Then suddenly you will no longer desire it. Liquorice really supports the adrenal glands. It takes over some of the functions, so that the gland can rest and recover from overuse.

The adrenal glands also regulate our blood pressure by producing a hormone called aldosterone. When the adrenal glands are exhausted, their output of aldosterone will be weak. The symptoms of low aldosterone levels are fatigue, salt-craving, "cognitive fuzziness", light-headedness upon standing, or palpitations with low blood pressure. The low levels of aldosterone means that the kidneys lose salt, leading to low blood volume.

Thus, one of the very best home treatments for adrenal fatigue is salt liquorice. The commercial salt liquorice contains ammonium chloride, so I suggest to my patients that they buy pure liquorice either as a juice stick or the root, and make a tea from this, then add a pinch of unrefined sea salt. This will marvellously support your adrenals, your blood pressure and your recovery.

## Angelica
## (*Angelica archangelica*)

The archangel of angels growing in our garden. A handsome herb which can easily grow in our climate, and is an underappreciated herb in my small opinion. If you look at the plant, you see a strong and strapping fellow, with a powerful energy field radiating around him. The root, herb and seeds can all be used, but I prefer to use the root.

Rich in volatile oils, it has an aromatic, warming quality to it, and has been used for centuries to restore vigour to the stomach and the lungs. Now if you think about it, we draw our vitality and nourishment from the food in our stomachs and the air we breathe. Both of these give us life, and this is why angelica is a strengthening herb, because it reinvigorates those organs, and is used for those who are so burnt out that they are cold within.

Sometimes when I speak to someone who is burned out, I see an image of a fire, where the coals have gone cold and there is just the hint of red amongst the grey ash. A vital and alive person has a strong fire. A person who is so depleted that their fire has gone out cannot bear anything too strong, just as you might imagine that throwing fire-lighting fluid on cold coals could very well extinguish the last sparks of light. Those coals need to be gently blown upon, with little kindling twigs before they can take on the big logs once again. People are the same; they need to be gently warmed and nourished, and so you can see why angelica is perfect.

Angelica has other benefits too. It kills off opportunistic bugs such as bacteria and viruses; warms the gut so that you can digest and absorb your nutrients again; and clears the lungs, so that you can draw breath. Which is what is needed – you need to stop, and draw breath.

## PEACE TEA

🍃 Make a blend of fragrant rose petals, lavender flowers, chamomile flowers, Californian poppy petals and lemon balm. Dry in a cool place and then store in an airtight container like a tea tin.

🍃 You can use 1 teaspoon of these lovely garden petals per cup of boiling water to make a refreshing and peace-inducing infusion to be taken hot or cold, with or without honey. You can also sweeten it a little with a dash of elderflower cordial.

## Porridge oats

Porridge oats are a very helpful herb for an overstimulated and depleted nervous system. People with this condition may describe themselves as feeling wired yet tired. As medical herbalists, we use fresh green oat kernels, which can easily be grown in your garden, and harvested when the kernel is still soft and squidgy. At this point, oats are referred to as milky oats, and the kernel can be tinctured and used as a tonic for an exhausted nervous system. If you prefer to avoid alcohol, then an oxymel (a mixture of honey and vinegar) would be a lovely method of preserving the milky-oat goodness. Having said all that, even when you eat a bowl of porridge oats, you instinctively can feel the nourishment that it gives you for they are rich in B vitamins, magnesium, iron, manganese, phosphorous, copper, zinc and potassium. I love to suggest oats for those people who are so very tired that they are trembling within. They are too tired to absorb their food. Porridge oats are soothing, healing, comforting and restorative.

One of the best times to eat oats is before you fall asleep. People with adrenal fatigue often struggle to fall asleep, or wake up during the night with a start and then can't sleep. This can be due to dropping blood sugar levels, which their exhausted body is unable to balance as it normally does. Oats give that slow-release carbohydrate support, along with natural B vitamins which calm and strengthen the nervous system.

*Even when you eat a bowl of porridge oats, you instinctively can feel the nourishment that it gives you for they are rich in B vitamins, magnesium, iron, manganese, phosphorous, copper, zinc and potassium.*

## BEDTIME OATS

Make a small bowl of porridge oats, and add a tablespoon of ground almonds, slices of half a banana, and a little butter. Loosening the porridge with a little almond milk will support your sleep. You don't need sugar because the banana will give the necessary sweetness as well as nutrients.

Almonds are rich in melatonin and magnesium which both facilitate a restful sleep. They also have protein and fat which delays the dropping of blood sugars.

Bananas are rich in magnesium and tryptophan, both of which encourage a good night's sleep. They are also rich in potassium which is important for nerve and muscle function.

The fat in the butter will slow the absorption of the porridge, helping to maintain your blood sugar levels during the night. Butter is also rich in butyric acid, which supports the health of the gut lining.

# Lettuce sleep

After his narrow escape from Mr McGregor, Peter Rabbit had a tummy ache and Mrs Josephine Rabbit sent him to bed with a cup of chamomile tea and a lettuce sandwich, which was very clever indeed.

The bitter white sap from lettuce contains a substance known as lactucarium (lettuce opium), which has a sedating effect on our minds, whilst the bitterness stimulates the secretion of digestive enzymes. After such a dreadful afternoon, he would have been in sympathetic-nervous-system dominance, which would have switched off the digestive enzymes but pushed the blood into his muscles so that he could flee.

This is not dissimilar to the way many of us live our lives – rushing around, lots of anxiety and suffering with irritable bowel syndrome (IBS) and small intestinal bacterial overgrowth (SIBO). Many of the underlying causes of those two conditions can be related back to stress on our nervous systems. Racing around in an overstimulated, adrenalized state is another reason why those with pre-burnout cannot digest their food properly. In order to properly digest your food, you need to be in the calm para-sympathetic state (rest and digest), which is our natural state. Being over-adrenalized puts us into the sympathetic-nervous state of fight or flight, and when we are in that state, our bodies divert blood from the digestive system to the muscles and heart in order to deal with the emergency. The secretion of enzymes is shut off, and food therefore cannot be digested.

Most people I have treated with adrenal fatigue are so very tired, and yet struggle to fall asleep. Wild lettuce (*Lactuca virosa*) is the herb which is used by medical herbalists, as it quietens overexcited tissues, but you can use romaine lettuce, which is also rich in the milky sap. Why not try a deeply filled lettuce sandwich and a cup of chamomile tea before bed for a gentle night's sleep?

## Sloes (*Prunus spinosa*)

Herbs fall in and out of fashion, and blackthorn has been out of fashion amongst medical herbalists for a long time. As such, there isn't much information about the plant, but it is known that ancient peoples used it, for pits near Glastonbury and in Switzerland were found to be full of the sloe pips. The berry is very bitter and astringent, but as we all know, soaked in alcohol, it makes a mellow warming drink. No doubt the ancients knew all about that.

When collecting sloes, for goodness' sake, do not collect on 11 November. This is the day of the Lunantishees, a race of Celtic faeries who live in the blackthorn tree. If you cut the tree on this day, bad luck will surely curse you. Rather, honour the faeries by tying a black ribbon about the trunk, and leave an offering of milk, cake and butter. I am sure that they will bless your sloe gin if you collect your berries the following day.

The Celtic name for blackthorn is "*straif*", from which our modern word "strife" is derived. Look carefully at this protective tree. It is a dark and tangled tree/shrub, impenetrable, and as such, a formidable hedge. Traditionally this tree either symbolizes that unavoidable strife is upon you, or it offers protection from this strife. This does not mean that the strife will not befall you, but if you can imagine yourself protected by a hedge of blackthorn, you are safe from the worst of the attack. Blackthorn is the first to flower after the long cold winter. It brings nectar to the tiny insects, which feed the birds, and so the dance of life begins again. Blackthorn flowers are a symbol of hope; the light in the dark. The torch of guidance that the worst is over, and your life can begin again. Thus blackthorn is the symbol of protection and hope.

The berries and the young shoots are used to make a medicine which is bursting with antioxidants and vitamin C. It has long been used as a tonic, in particular for those who feel exhausted and sluggish following a bacterial or viral infection. I would use this herb for someone suffering from post-viral fatigue.

It is a deeply cleansing herb, and I would consider it very useful for supporting the heart, specifically when pericarditis is the result of a viral infection. Quite often with fatigue and anxiety, you will find the person suffers from palpitations and trembling. This herb, combined with hawthorn and motherwort, will calm the palpitations and give strength to the exhausted heart.

*♪ ♪ ♪*

There are many wonderful herbs to treat fatigue, but I do beg you to see a medical herbalist. There are so many things to consider with someone who is burned out: the immune system, the adrenals, the nervous system, their digestive function. This is really best considered on a one-to-one basis.

## NUTRIENT-DENSE FOODS

For the chronically fatigued person, we return to the nourishing soup which I described at the beginning of the book – sometimes people are so depleted of their vital force that they literally cannot digest and absorb their food.

The calorific energy required to digest and absorb nutrients from our food is referred to as the thermic effect. On average, our bodies use between 10–30 per cent of our energy digesting. Some people just don't have enough energy, and for these folk, their ability to absorb the nutrients required to run their body is much impaired.

It is useful to consider the thermic effect of different foods. Fats only require 3 per cent of the energy that they provide. Vegetables and fruit require 20 per cent, and proteins require 30 per cent. So, you can see that foods rich in protein would benefit from long cooking, for instance as a soup or casserole, because this helps to soften the protein and make it more digestible. Fats in the meal soothe the digestive tract and provide energy for the depleted person. Vegetables and fruits, of course, provide the vitamins and minerals; however, I always suggest to my exhausted patients that well-cooked food will be far more profitable than cold raw foods like salads, until they strengthen. An exhausted person is cold, therefore they need warm, soft and easily digestible foods to restore their health. Once they have regained some strength then they can include raw, nutrient-rich foods like avocados and salads.

In order to avoid overwhelming the digestive system, it helps to eat little and often, small but highly nourishing meals. Some of the suggestions below require time in the kitchen, and others are much simpler, but the cooking process can be used as a creative me-time moment. If cooking is too much for you, then good-quality ready meals with fresh vegetables are a decent option until you are able to cook again.

**Examples of easily digestible and nourishing meals include:**

- Chicken, mushroom and vegetable soup made from nourishing bone broth stock. Of course, if you are vegetarian then you would rather use a rich shiitake mushroom and root vegetable stock.

- Scrambled eggs and spinach.

- Soft boiled eggs on spinach or good-quality toast, with butter.

- Casseroles with mashed root vegetables such as swede, celeriac, sweet potato or parsnips, and other vegetables of your choice.

- Smoked salmon or mackerel, steamed new potatoes with butter, and baby tomatoes with avocado salad.

- Fish and mashed potato with good butter, and some vegetables; or fish pie.

- Roasted butternut, onions and mushrooms on a bed of steamed and buttered kale, or mashed root vegetables.

- Meat or vegetarian sausages with mashed sweet potato and green beans.

- Paleo cakes, like sweet-potato brownies, for a little treat.

- Porridge with banana and nutmeg.

- Dal with softly sauteed courgette (zucchini) and onions.

- Gentle vegetable curry cooked with coconut milk on basmati rice.

- Smoothies rich in nutritional foods such as blueberries, spinach, avocado, coconut, seasonal fruit, half a banana, even some nut butter. Add a tablespoon of chia seeds to cleanse your bowel.

- Basmati rice cooked in bone broth or chicken stock with soft steamed vegetables is helpful if you feel very tender in your stomach and have difficulty digesting food.

To support the digestive process, fresh pineapple and papaya provide natural digestive enzymes, and a small portion of either or both may be taken just before eating.

I find that people with adrenal fatigue cannot maintain their blood sugar levels, and quite often, they don't even realize that their blood sugars are low. When this happens, it puts the body back into a state of emergency, which is further exhausting to the body. For this reason, it is better to eat little and often so that you maintain your blood sugar balance. If you do this, you will immediately feel like you are on sturdier ground. You will feel a sense of strength, and will be more able to cope with your day. Simple snacks like almond butter on an oat biscuit, soup in a thermos flask, half an avocado, a bit of cold chicken, or hummus and carrots will just see you through to the next proper meal.

## NUTRITIONAL SUPPLEMENTS

Stress burns up nutrients, and nutritionists find that three nutritional supplements are particularly helpful. These include magnesium, vitamin C and vitamin B complex. My preferred choice is liquid magnesium (because it is so much more easily absorbed), liposomal vitamin C and a good-quality B complex. Again, I say that it is better to consult a nutritionist who can prescribe the correct nutrients for you. This is just a general idea.

People who have been stressed for a long time are usually low in magnesium, which gives rise to symptoms such as jumpy legs, difficulty falling asleep and muscle cramps. A wonderful adjunct to the magnesium supplements is to take an Epsom salt bath, or at the very least an Epsom salt foot bath, which you can enjoy whilst watching a gentle film, meditating or stroking the cat. Adding essential oils to the Epsom salts gives an added relaxing dimension to your home therapy. The dose is always two handfuls of Epsom salts per bath.

## RELAXING EPSOM SALT BATH OR FOOT BATH

2 handfuls of Epsom salts

12 drops of lavender essential oil

6 drops of Roman chamomile essential oil or 12 drops of lavender essential oil

8 drops of peppermint or rosemary essential oil (do not use rosemary if you are epileptic)

Add the salts to a glass or ceramic bowl, then drip the oils on top of the salts. Stir with a balloon whisk, and store in a glass jar until needed.

Run your bath, and just before you get in, add all the fragrant salts. The essential oils will immediately rise with the steam, so to enjoy their fragrance, close the bathroom door.

For a foot bath, add half the amount of fragrant salts to a bowl of water. You can cover your legs and feet with a thick towel to enhance the beneficial effects. You will still be able to enjoy the fragrant essential oils.

*The essential oils will immediately rise with the steam, so to enjoy their fragrance, close the bathroom door.*

# SOLFEGGIO MUSIC

The solfeggio tones are said to have originated in the 11th century through an Italian monk called Guido of Arezzo. These tones, which are vibrational frequencies, penetrate into our conscious and subconscious minds, as well as our cellular tissues.

Our bodies vibrate with electromagnetic waves at certain frequencies. When our cells and minds are exposed to vibrations, they oscillate together and can affect us. This is why we may be attracted or repelled by the energy in a room, or why sound can heal.

Humans (and no doubt plants and animals) respond positively to these sound vibrations, and certain frequencies can generate particular effects, so that you can choose your music to suit what it is that you want to resonate with.

**There are nine solfeggio frequencies:**

- **174Hz** – Considered to be a natural anaesthetic and healing to the organs. Removes physical and emotional pain.

- **285Hz** – Promotes the healing of damaged tissues. Said to be connected to our blueprint for optimal health.

- **396Hz** – Freedom from negative emotions; reduces fear, grief and anxiety. Helps to ground and restabilize the person.

- **417Hz** – Slows down the heart and promotes a feeling of peace and wellbeing. Transforms broken situations, cleanses traumatic situations.

- **528Hz** – Has a healing effect on the body, whilst at the same time reduces stress in the nervous and hormonal systems. It is said to repair DNA.

- **639Hz** – Balances the emotions and promotes communication, love, harmony and understanding between persons.

- **741Hz** – Helps with problem solving, promotes intuition and the awakening of your inner creativity. This frequency nurtures the will to live simply and in resonance with your inner truth. In other words, helps your brainwaves to become attuned to following your heart.

- **852Hz** – Dissolves the energy blockages which hinder self-realization. Helps to bring inner strength where you replace negative thoughts with positive ones. In that way you learn to live according to your higher ideals.

- **963Hz** – Activates the pineal gland and is associated with awakening intuition and our connection to source.

These pleasing non-intrusive sounds can be played as background music in your home to reharmonize your whole being and that of the home environment. They restore the electromagnetic vibrational fields of your brain and heart back into a healthy co-ordinated frequency, in tune with our natural Earth resonance. To access this music, you can find a wide variety available on the internet, through websites such as Relax Melodies.

# COMING HOME TO YOURSELF

Recovering from adrenal burnout is a journey, which can be painful, but it is wonderful too. It is quite possible that you will lose aspects of your life which you think are valuable but are probably no longer supporting you, or which are taking more than they give. You may lose people who you thought were friends, and gain friendships from those you never imagined would care.

I have twice burned out, and I clearly remember one time when I was weak, I kept getting images of myself as a snake shedding its skin. For months this image would float into my mind, and indeed, there were aspects of my life which had to be shed. Three very significant people dominated my life with their moods, and I had lost all contact with who I was. For weeks and months, this image worked on me. Of course, in the fullness of time, those people and aspects of my life fell away. Some of it was painful, but it was necessary, and was required for me to find my strength again, and to fully experience who I am without the influence of others clouding the scene.

You can let go with honour. You can be grateful for either the goodness that you once had from those aspects, or for the lessons learned from those aspects of your life which you no longer need, but try to let go with gratitude rather than with hate, because the energy of gratitude is healing. It's a good energy to carry. Let go of that which is outworn, but let it go with love, then you can set about enriching your life.

From a mental/emotional and even spiritual perspective, recovering from adrenal fatigue is all about bringing the richness that you deserve into your life, appreciating what life has to offer you, and what you want to offer life. It's living life to the full in a way that is sustainable and nourishing to your body, mind and spirit. Following your heart, your higher intuition, and living with joy.

Physically, recovering from fatigue is about doing things which nourish you but are not over-exerting. Yin yoga, meditation and mindfulness bring you back into the moment, and back to a state of peace. Walking in the forest, baking a cake, sewing a special garment, crafting something with wood, growing and harvesting your own food, writing a book – these all bring you into the moment, back down to Earth.

Many people don't know anything but work, and they don't have hobbies or know what they like to do with their time. In those cases, it is helpful to think back to yourself as a child. What did you love doing? Or, what did you wish you could do? When I was young, I loved horses, but I was also terrified of them, to the point that I would give them an apple, but only by tossing it over the fence onto the ground for them. I wouldn't feed them from my hand. When I was 24, I decided to learn to ride a horse. Now, I love them and am not afraid of those beautiful creatures, even though they are huge. I love to kiss wild horses, and I stand in awe of their gentleness and power, as they turned an aspect of my life into a treasure.

# CHAPTER 2

## Imbolc

Imagine yourself in those long and far-off days, when people lived close to the land. So close that you felt the numbing icy earth through your leathered shoes, the hollow-bellied pinch of starvation over winter, the sorrow of grief for those lost to illnesses during the shivering months, and then the relief when the Sun God and the Earth Mother worked their annual magic, drawing life once again up through the frozen soil. As the days grow longer, and the first shy hints of life peep up at the pale sun, it doesn't feel like it yet, but new life is already in the air.

The Celtic celebration of Imbolc occurs on 1 February, the mid-point between the Winter Solstice and the Spring Equinox. The word "Imbolc" variously derives from Old Irish or Proto-Indo-European, meaning "in milk", or "in the belly", referring to the time of year when the ewes are pregnant and beginning to lactate. Now a rich supply of fat and protein becomes available for milk and cheese, which will be eaten with the new spring greens, restoring life force and vigour to the hungry land.

Brigid is the goddess associated with Imbolc. She is a goddess of smithcraft, poetry and healing. She is the exalted one, represented by the purity of white snow, and associated with high ideals and morals, but also with sacred wells, cleansing and healing. To celebrate Imbolc, you may choose to go on a pilgrimage, seeking out wells sacred to Brigid. Or, perhaps you might build a little well in your garden or home to honour her. Fill a glass or clay bowl with some spring water and surround it with moss, snowdrops and green or white candles to represent the sun, new growth and the purity of your intentions. You might even like to add a little sheep's wool found caught on thorny hedges to welcome in the bouncing lambs soon to be born.

You could begin your ceremony by calling her name and then tossing a coin into the water. Stare at the ripples as you ask for creative inspiration, or her blessings on your endeavours. Wash your fingers in the well as a symbol of cleansing away illness, or write her a poem from your heart. Light the candles as a symbol of hope for the Earth, embody her as a goddess of life by feeding little birds during this difficult time of the year for them, plant trees to replenish the land, or a bed of flowers for the bees and butterflies.

# NOOTROPICS – HERBS FOR THE BRAIN

### 🌿 CHOCOLATE 🌿 NETTLE SEEDS 🌿 SAGE
### 🌿 ROSEMARY 🌿 TURMERIC 🌿 PERIWINKLE

Imbolc represents the growing light in darkest days, and from this we may take the liberty of expanding the concept to our own bright sparks – our brains. There is a class of smart drugs known as nootropics, which help to improve mental functions such as focus, memory, creativity and motivation. Nootropics may be helpful for sufferers of Alzheimer's or Parkinson's disease, but are particularly useful for those who have had a tough time and feel less mentally sharp than they used to. This is commonly referred to as "brain fog", where you just cannot think clearly. It is as if you have cotton wool in your head and you become forgetful, you can't focus and sometimes your brain hurts. This often happens as a result of illness. Nootropics can also be very helpful at times when you need to study intensively, or sometimes we are just getting on in life and the little grey cells aren't what they used to be.

Always start by nourishing yourself with your food. It may surprise you to discover that gluten sensitivity is much more common than we think. The symptoms may not always present as bloating, diarrhoea and flatulence as we had previously thought, but more common and hidden symptoms include insulin resistance, poor memory, brain fog and headaches.[13] [14] Of equal importance is to cut out the dangerous trans-fats which you find in fried foods and margarines, and a big one: radically reduce your sugar intake.

The foods which really feed the brain are healthy fats, in particular, the omega-3 fatty acids derived from oily fish such as mackerel, salmon and sardines. Vegetable options include flaxseeds, chia and hemp seeds, walnuts and soya beans. Look at the shape of the walnut – it says it all! Other healthy fats include eggs, avocados and coconut oil.

The simplest way to eat well, is to imagine what a caveman might have eaten. They didn't eat a lot of grains, but ate fish and meat, nuts and seeds, lots of fruit, vegetables and roots. By eating organically, you avoid putting insecticides and hormones into your body, whilst at the same time helping to support a healthy environment both on the Earth and in your intestines.

# NOOTROPICS

The word "nootropic" originates from two Greek words. "Noo" is derived from the Greek word "*nous*", which refers to your mind or intellect.

The second part of the word, "tropic", is derived from "*tropikos*", and means "turning toward", or "affecting the activity of". Thus, nootropics are substances which affect the mind. Nootropics are defined as a class of substances, both synthetic and natural, which enhance cognition, memory, focus, attention and alertness, facilitate learning and can improve mood. We are going to focus on natural nootropics which can easily be found in your kitchen or garden and of which scientific studies have confirmed their traditional uses.

## Chocolate

The wonderful news is that chocolate can really boost your mental health, both in terms of mood and cognition. The caveat is that it needs to be of a high cocoa content, raw if possible and low in sugar. However, the benefits are sweet.

It is worth differentiating between cocoa and cacao. Cocoa is the normal cocoa powder where the beans have been roasted and powdered. The nutritional value is less (but not lacking) when compared to cacao, which has been fermented and processed at much lower temperatures.

The cocoa bean provides us with a magical concoction of natural chemicals which make you feel amazing, all wrapped up in a package of delicious darkness. No wonder it is called the food of the gods. I make sure that I eat it every day. I eat 90 per cent cocoa solids, which I understand is too much for most people, but it is low in sugar and has a rich flavour which means that just two squares daily is satisfying.

Enrobed in cacao is a gentle stimulant called theobromine, which dilates the blood vessels, increasing blood flow to the brain. In doing so, extra nutrition is delivered to the brain cells, enhancing cognition. The improved blood flow also delivers the other amazing natural chemicals found in chocolate, such as a rich range of flavonoids.

These, too, improve blood flow to the brain, promoting the development of nerve connections, especially in the areas of the brain involved with learning and memory, and some studies have found that cocoa can lower the risk of developing Alzheimer's disease.[15] Whilst all cells must die, we don't want them to die before their time, and the flavonoids found in chocolate, dark-skinned fruits and vegetables help to protect our brain cells from early death, as well as promoting the connectivity between brain cells. Our creativity and mental clarity depend upon good connectivity between healthy brain cells. This connectivity supports long-term memory formation, improves focus, attention, processing speed and cognition.[16]

Phenylethylamine (PEA) in chocolate helps to increase another chemical called tyrosine, which in turn develops into dopamine, resulting in increased sensations of pleasure and reward. Now PEA in itself is rather wonderful. Remember how boxes of chocolates so often play a part in the courting rituals of couples? Well, dark unprocessed chocolate is rich in PEA, often referred to as the love molecule because it increases that feeling of being in lurve!

Chocolate is also rich in tryptophan, the precursor of serotonin which is known as our happy hormone. This neurotransmitter raises our mood and decreases our appetite. Those people who eat when they are feeling low may be lacking in serotonin.

We find another chemical in chocolate called anandamide, which is commonly referred to as the bliss chemical, because it banishes anxiety and reduces pain sensations. It almost takes us to a heavenly place in our minds. Black pepper, which contains the alkaloid guineesine, blocks the breakdown of anandamide, thereby increasing or prolonging its blissful effects.

◦ ◦ ◦

## BLACK PEPPER HOT CHOCOLATE

This delicious hot chocolate is really warming, but it is great for boosting your mood and brain power too. I would consider this a jolly nice consolation prize for those who have to study on cold wintry days.

240ml (1 cup) coconut milk
1 tsp coconut oil
1 tsp cacao powder
stevia or xylitol
grind of black pepper

Warm the coconut milk, then whisk the coconut oil and cacao powder into the milk. Sweeten to taste, and stir in a generous amount of freshly ground black pepper.

# Nettle seeds (*Urtica dioica*)

Nettle seeds are a treasure trove hidden in plain sight. Within those little green clusters of seeds lie a superfood waiting to provide you with lusty vigour. The seeds hold fatty acids 3, 6 and 9, giving not only the brain but the cardiac system a nice boost of omegas.

We all know that nettles contain histamine, the chemical that is responsible for the sting, and you will probably not be surprised to note that histamine acts as an excitatory chemical, stimulating arousal in the brain and the whole body.

Now this is interesting, because there goes a story that the doctor in charge of an old-age care home insisted that the nurses put 1 teaspoon of nettle seeds on the residents' morning porridge. Apparently, they became "lusty". It is not elaborated on whether this was in song or behaviour, but the nettle seeds certainly perked up their petals.

This is why herbalists use nettle seeds. It is specifically indicated for those who feel tired, jaded and worn out. The seeds are particularly used for those who experience what you might call "brain fatigue". In the spring, we use the young leaves because they provide a good boost of minerals and vitamins, as well as acting as a blood cleanser, which is what we need after stodgy winter food. But in the winter months, we need nourishment of a different kind. We need healthy fats and a tonic to get us through the cold, dark days.

The easiest way to collect the seeds is to wait until the end of summer, when you will see bright green clusters of seeds hanging from the old nettles. Snip the nettle stem to about a third of the way down and gather your stems into bundles, then tie them with string. Place them head down inside a paper bag and hang to dry in a warm place. From time to time, give the head of stems a good shake, and you will find that the seeds drop neatly into the bag. Once you are sure that you have collected all the seeds, you can burn the stems, and spread the ash over your vegetables or roses.

Take 1 teaspoon daily on your porridge. But do sieve and rub the seeds well in a cloth to break the little itchy hairs. Enjoy your lusty health.

## BRAINY NETTLE SEED AND WALNUT CHOCOLATE

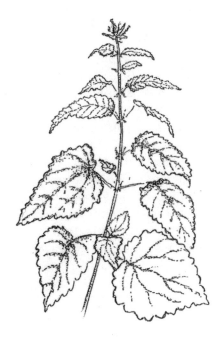

🌿 Break up a bar of very dark chocolate into a saucepan and place this in a frying pan which has been filled with water, so that you form a bain-marie. Melt the chocolate.

🌿 In the meantime, roughly chop your walnuts, then stir them into your chocolate.

🌿 Now pour the melted chocolate onto a piece of greaseproof (waxed) paper and quickly sprinkle liberally with nettle seeds and goji berries. Allow to cool, then snap into small pieces and store in a cake tin.

## Sage (*Salvia officinalis*)

Sage did not get its name for nothing. It might be sage advice to drink it if you want to preserve your brain power, especially as you get older. This herb has long been valued for its ability to enhance cognition, improve memory, quicken the senses and delay age-associated cognitive deterioration, and now, human studies confirm that sage offers significant cognitive improvements in persons suffering from symptoms of Alzheimer's.[17]

Studies show that sage helps to inhibit the accumulation of the amyloid-β peptide, which is significant in the development of Alzheimer's disease. In particular, it is the rosmarinic acids which do this job, and clearly, these constituents are also present in rosemary too, another "brain herb".[18]

Sage, and nettle seeds too for that matter, help to prevent the breakdown of an important neurotransmitter called acetylcholine. In doing so, they contribute toward the preservation of memory, attention, learning and motivation. In other words, these herbs help to keep you "bright".

Sage also shows a powerful free-radical scavenging property, which is very important in maintaining cognitive function. It reduces anxiety and defends against depression, and drinking sage brings about an enhancement of alertness, calmness and contentedness.

The time of collection and the method of extraction of the constituents which provide the benefits is important. The best times for collection are May, July and September, and the best method of extraction is an alcoholic extraction.

My suggestion is that you collect your leaves in May and July, and stuff them into a Kilner jar with vodka, brandy or gin because you need at least 40 per cent alcohol. Leave to macerate for 2 weeks, then strain and bottle. Take 1 teaspoon daily. If you can't take alcohol, simply drop one or two leaves in a teapot of boiling water (a teapot is important because you don't want to allow those valuable volatile oils to vaporize away), then enjoy as your daily brainy cuppa.

## Rosemary (*Rosmarinus officinalis*)

Shakespeare said it when he wrote, "There's rosemary, that's for remembrance." It has ever been thus. Since ancient Egypt, the herb has been used in funeral ceremonies to preserve and remember the deceased, and ancient Greek students would circle garlands of it upon their heads to facilitate their memories. Stroke the plant and the tangy aroma will immediately lift your spirits. It is one of our most beloved herbs with many more uses than memory, but for now, that is what we are focusing on.

Very similarly to sage, it defends against Alzheimer's disease, and possibly Parkinson's disease, by protecting the neurons and restraining amyloid plaque formation. For younger people, studies show that vaporized rosemary essential oil significantly improves short-term memory. After inhaling the essential oil, they reported feeling mentally fresher.[19] Another study showed that inhaled rosemary essential oil increased blood pressure, respiratory rate and heart rate so that the sample group were stimulated into a more alert state. Rosemary changes our brainwaves from the quiet and restful alpha state to the problem-solving beta waves, where we are attentive and focused.[20]

An interesting study compared the effects of rosemary with peppermint and lavender essential oils. In accordance with tradition, the rosemary and peppermint improved short-term memory of the group, whilst the lavender worsened it but made everyone feel calm and relaxed.[21] However, to be focused, you need to feel calm, so a combination of all three would make a great blend to vaporize in the office.

All three herbs can be taken as a tea, but I think they are nicest when their essential oils are vaporized in the room where you need to focus.

**CAUTION:** Rosemary should not be used in any way if you have had seizures, as it may trigger a seizure.

## REFRESHING STUDY BLEND

4 drops of rosemary essential oil
2 drops of peppermint essential oil
2 drops of lavender essential oil, and/
    or 2 drops of lemon essential oil

Add this blend of oils to a diffuser to freshen the room and your brain.

## CALMING AND UPLIFTING BLEND

This is a lovely blend when you feel tired, and want to feel quietly alert.

4 drops of rosemary essential oil
4 drops of lavender essential oil
3 drops of sweet orange essential oil

For instance, after a busy day at work, this makes a gentle evening refresher blend, either in your bath or diffused in the air of the kitchen. If the weather is very hot, you may prefer to swap the rosemary for peppermint.

## BRAIN SPICE

Spice up your food and your brain with this homemade condiment, which drip-feeds your brain with nootropic herbs.

5 tbsp sea salt crystals
1 tsp nettle seeds
1 tsp dried and crushed sage leaves
1 tsp dried and crushed rosemary
    leaves
1 tsp turmeric powder
¼ tsp ground black pepper

Mix all the ingredients together and add to a salt grinder, so that every day you freshly grind these lovely healing condiments onto your food.

## Turmeric (*Curcuma longa*)

Turmeric is the great protector. With its amazing antioxidant and anti-inflammatory actions, this root is able to protect against the ravages of ageing on our minds as well as our joints, whilst at the same time helping to fight depression. Brain-derived neurotrophic factor (BDNF) is a natural chemical in our body, which facilitates the growth of new nerves and protects nerves against oxidative damage, and in doing so, is much involved in the formation, retention and recall of memory. People who are overweight or diabetic have been found to have low levels of BDNF, but curcumin, a major constituent found in turmeric, helps to correct this.[22]

Turmeric doesn't only preserve our youthful intellect but also our joints, plus it protects us from cancer, heals our gut lining and no doubt has a catalogue of other benefits which we are yet to learn about. Turmeric loves to work with coconut oil, as the people of India well know. Coconut oil is rich in medium-chain fatty acids, which boost brain function and memory, lower blood sugar levels, and aid weight loss and energy levels.

## Periwinkle (*Vinca minor*)

Periwinkle is another of those gorgeous herbs so often forgotten nowadays. It loves to ramble happily along the forest floor under the shade of trees and shrubs, where its flowers throw the most beautiful shades of violet for our eyes to savour.

Violet is the colour of the crown chakra, and it is indeed the head and the nervous system which is so positively affected by periwinkle. The leaves and flowers of *Vinca minor*, when taken as a medicine, literally open the brain. The plant contains an alkaloid called vincamine, which dilates the blood vessels in our brain, thus enhancing cerebral blood flow.[23]

Another alkaloid found in *Vinca minor* known as vincamine is of particular interest for scientists in relation to strokes, where the brain damage is caused by the oxygen deprivation of the stroke. This constituent enhances blood flow and has neuroprotective effects on the brain.[24]

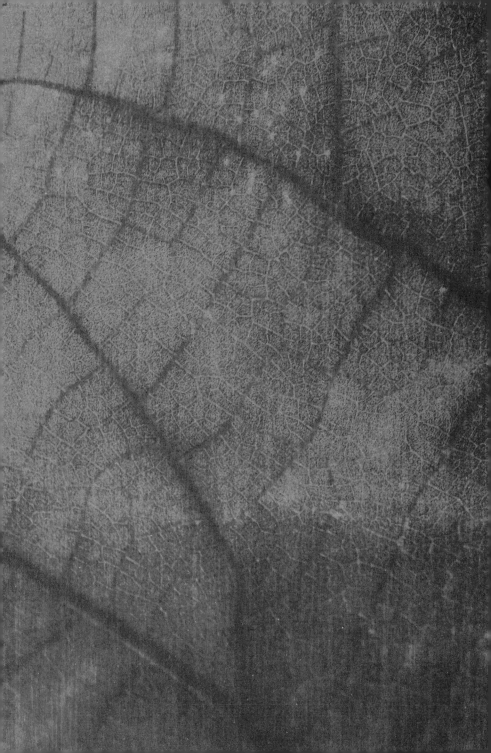

# CHAPTER 3

## Spring Equinox

# SPRING –
# THE TURNING OF THE YEAR

*BIRCH * NETTLE * GROUND ELDER
*BURDOCK * CLIVERS * CHICKWEED * HORSETAIL

On 19, 20 and 21 March in the northern hemisphere, the Earth's equator tips to an angle that is perpendicular to the sun's rays. This means that there is almost exactly an equal amount of light as there is dark in a 24-hour period. The equinox marks the beginning of springtime up here, or autumn if you are in the southern hemisphere. Winter releases its ice-fast grip, and we all start to relax a little as we enjoy the growing warmth of the sun.

This is a time of balance, where darkness gives way to the light. It is a time when we can contemplate the balance within our own lives. Perhaps time to start venturing outdoors a bit more, engaging with nature as the plants of the land gather momentum in their reaching upward toward the light.

The surge of the rising tree sap is discernible, not least so in the beautiful birch, whose sap has been harvested at this time of year for centuries, especially in the far north. Those harvesters turn the sap into wine, mead, vinegar and syrup. It is used as a medicine and valued as a beauty product.

*This is a time of balance, where darkness gives way to the light. It is a time when we can contemplate the balance within our own lives.*

# BIRCH –
# THE TREE OF NEW BEGINNINGS

According to the Celtic Ogham tree calendar, the birch tree is placed in January/February because she symbolizes new beginnings and a fresh start. I have placed her at the Spring Equinox, because that is when her sap begins to rise and she starts to wake from her winter stillness, transforming into the fullness of her elegant summer form. There are few visions as breathtaking to behold as a grove of birch trees, swaying together in a quiet moonlit forest. It is a vision of grace, whispering of another dimension in our world, where trees and faeries dance under a full moon to the shimmer of the breeze and an orchestra of frogs.

## THE BEAUTIFUL LADY

Throughout the northern hemisphere, she is so renowned for her gracefulness, radiance in the moonlight and flowing suppleness stirred by the air, that she has been called the Beautiful Lady, the Shining Tree or the White Lady of the Woods. In Russia, they love this tree as a goddess. There, the beauty of a young lady is often compared with that of a birch, suggesting that she is graceful and slim like a young birch tree. Indeed, these qualities also describe the therapeutic benefits which she confers upon those who know.

In the Russian taiga forest, the tree is hailed as white gold, because of the beneficial effects it has on skin conditions such as eczema, psoriasis and even skin cancers. The whiteness of her bark comes from a constituent called betulin. This is also found in the birch sap, which is tapped around the second week of March, and is taken as a cleansing and healing tonic water. Betulin has many therapeutic actions such as antibacterial and anti-inflammatory properties, alleviating itchiness and promoting the regeneration of hair and healthy skin tissue. It may even induce cancer cells to die.[25]

Betulin reduces obesity and cholesterol, and increases cellular sensitivity to insulin in those who are carrying too much weight. The bark, also being rich in salicylates, relieves the inflammation of stiff and arthritic joints, whilst the leaves help to flush out the acid crystals which cause the stiffness. With all these marvellous properties being transferred to us from the beautiful birch, we too can enjoy the same supple grace as she, if we will only imbibe her abundant gifts.

Growing on her bark, and looking for all the world just like a dark tumour itself, grows the amazing chaga mushroom, which the Russians call "the diamond in the forest". It is well documented as a superfood which both prevents and may suppress cancer tumour growth, if taken as a tea daily.[26] Like its host, this strange-looking fungus is rich in betulinic acid and other beneficial compounds, and also helps to facilitate weight loss, reduce cholesterol and blood sugar levels, and boost the immune system.

Observe for a moment the shape of the tree. See how her leaves appear to flow like a waterfall? The long tendrils swaying in the breeze suggest a few more clues to us. She is indeed a watery tree of flow. In the springtime, birch tappers are able to harvest on average five litres of sap a day from each tree. Her leaves are diuretic, and flush the toxins out of our bodies by increasing our watery flow. The antibacterial, antiviral and antifungal action of the leaves, with the diuretic and anti-inflammatory actions, makes an infusion of leaves a very effective first aid remedy for kidney infections, cystitis and even kidney gravel when drunk over a long period of time.

She offers more. She is a beauty product. The leaves, traditionally used to reduce weight and cellulite, are also rich in vitamin C, which helps to build collagen, thereby plumping up wrinkles and sagging skin.

As an excellent hair tonic, you can rub the leftover tea from your teapot directly to the scalp, for the leaves strengthen hair and stimulate the growth. These leaves are also rich in soapy saponins, which gently cleanse the hair and soothe an irritated scalp, all this making the birch a helpful friend to those who have lost their hair after childbirth, chemotherapy or following stressful periods in their lives. So, immediately we see how the beauty of the tree reflects the beauty which it bestows upon those who drink of her goodness. And yet, this abundant goddess of the woods gives us even more gifts.

# BIRCH AS A MEDICINE

Bark and roots are always the most difficult parts of the plant to use, partly because they are hard work to access, but mainly because you stand a great chance of killing the plant, which would be horrible. Bark and roots can be purchased from suppliers who know how to harvest sustainably, so that the tree or plant is not killed. Leaves, flowers and buds are easy to harvest, and in the case of birch, quite safe, unless you are allergic to salicylates or aspirin.

**CAUTION:** Do not use birch in any form if you are allergic to aspirin or salicylates. If you are taking blood-thinning medication, it is fine to use birch topically, but not internally.

## BIRCH-BUD TEA

To help with urinary tract infection, it would be best to use the leaf buds. These can be collected in springtime, and dried in the shade, then stored in a paper bag.

Use 1 teaspoon per cup of boiling water. Steep for 10 minutes in a teapot, or in a cup with a saucer on top, then drink 4 cups daily. If your symptoms don't resolve within 3 days, do see your doctor or a medical herbalist.

So, immediately we see how the beauty of the tree reflects the beauty which it bestows upon those who drink of her goodness.

## BIRCH HAIR TONIC

**A hair tonic can be made in the same manner as the birch-bud tea, but in this case, you would use slightly older leaves rather than buds.**

🍂 Pick the leaves in late spring or early summer. You may choose to add some rosemary to stimulate circulation to the scalp, or horsetail herb to strengthen the hair shaft, or both!

🍂 Add equal quantities of all herbs, and dry in the usual way, in a cool area out of the sun so as not to spoil the rosemary in particular. When dry, I would crush the leaves with my hands, so that they are smaller and mix together more easily.

🍂 To make the tonic, add 1 tablespoon of your herbal mixture to a teapot of boiling water. Steep for an hour before you use it, then strain. Now add 1 tablespoon of apple cider vinegar, and pour over your hair daily as a hair tonic, or as a final rinse after shampooing. Don't rinse out, just dry in the usual way.

## BIRCH-LEAF OIL

**For skin conditions, you can make a birch-leaf oil. The oil you choose should also be therapeutic, so you might like to choose something healing like jojoba, coconut or macadamia nut oil.**

🍂 Collect the leaves in springtime and, making sure that they are not wet with dew or rain, push them into a wide-neck jar, then top up with the oil of your choice. I don't find that leaving leaves in oil on a sunny windowsill is warm enough to extract the constituents from the leaves, and so I prefer to use a bain-marie.

🍂 To do this, you place some warm water in a frying pan, then a small saucepan with your leaves and oil is placed into the water-bath frying pan. Now switch on the hob so that the heat warms the water and this gently warms the oil. This should be done while you are in the kitchen and takes about an hour or two.

When the oil has turned a deep shade of green, you take the saucepan out of the watery bath and allow the oil to cool. Strain through a clean muslin cloth, then add a few drops of geranium essential oil to preserve the oil.

Bottle your birch oil, and keep in the refrigerator or a cool dark cupboard until you need it.

This birch oil is effective for skin conditions such as eczema, psoriasis, aching joints and cellulite.

## BIRCH-LEAF OINTMENT FOR ACHING JOINTS
**You might find it less messy to turn your oil into an ointment.**

To do this, you need to warm 50ml (1¾fl oz) of the oil gently in a bain-marie, then add 1 heaped teaspoon of beeswax peas (tiny consolidated drops of beeswax) and allow the wax to melt.

You might like to strengthen your ointment – if so, add 20 drops of birch essential oil to the bottom of a 60ml (2fl oz) glass jar, then pour the hot ointment over it. Now quickly close the lid to prevent the essential oil from vaporizing.

## BIRCH AND CYPRESS CELLULITE SALT

Add 2 handfuls of fine sea salt to a glass jar which can be sealed.

Add 20 drops of cypress essential oil to the salt, and shake thoroughly so that the oil is well distributed in the jar.

Now add as much of your birch oil as is needed so that the salt is covered by 1cm (½in).

Use this medicated salt to vigorously rub any areas with cellulite to shift the congestion. Rinse it off in the shower, or enjoy the therapeutic benefits in a bath.

## PHYTONCIDES IN THE FOREST

She is a killer. Rich in phytoncides, the volatile aromatic oils of forest wood, the birch tree kills those who seek to attack her.

Rather chillingly, the word "phytoncides" means "death by plant". There are 5,000 odd volatile substances used by forest trees to kill the insects, bacteria or fungi which would otherwise eat or rot the tree, and as such, they are also powerful cleansers of the air. When the air within a birch forest is measured for microbes, it is found to hold fewer germs than would normally be found in a modern sterile operating theatre.[27]

But to us, phytoncides are friendly and have beneficial effects on our health. One study showed that they markedly increase our immune system's natural killer cells, whilst at the same time reduce our adrenaline (epinephrine) – the very hormone which squashes our immune response.[28]

A few years ago, you used to be considered, at best, a bit odd if you tree-hugged; at worst, highly suspicious if you were seen loitering in the forest without a dog or any other plausible excuse. But now, in these more enlightened times, forest bathing has become a common recreation, and scientists are even studying its effect on our health. Lo, they have found that those who spend time in forests have significantly improved immune systems, are happier and less depressed for days after the forest experience.

## THE WITCH'S BROOMSTICK

Even as an adult, I remain disappointed that witches do not go hurtling through the stormy night skies on their broomsticks. However, the witches' besoms, made from birch twigs, do have another magical purpose. On a mundane level, they sweep away dust, wood ash and leaves from the home. In Russia, the birch is venerated as a gift from God, given to them for protection, and they believe that the birch should be planted near the house so that the birch spirit may guard against all evil forces.

On a magical level, the birch besom is used for cleansing away that which is no longer necessary in our lives, because you cannot welcome in new energy when old stuff is cluttering up your life. Just like an over-full bookshelf.

In the past, birch twigs have been used to sweep away "evil energies". Today we might refer to this as recurring negative thoughts, old unwanted energies, possibly even banishing troublesome people from our lives. So, we might use birch symbolically to cleanse our life field of negative influences, or sweep just above the head to clear the channels between the divine and the crown chakra so that we may "hear" the inspiration more clearly. Using trees or plants symbolically is not a waste of time. By taking the time to enact the symbolic ritual, you send a powerful message to your subconscious mind. That part of the mind runs 95 per cent of our life choices, so it has power. Having said that, magic does work. It has worked in my life, and that of many of my friends, so please, do get out your broomsticks. One thing that is extremely important – never use magic to harm anyone.

You too could make your own besom from birch twigs, bound around a birch branch to symbolically sweep away the energy of anything that you want to be free of, so that you can make space for fresh new beginnings at the start of the new year. Or, you might choose to bind birch twigs around a hazel staff, for hazel is the tree of inspiration. In that way, you sweep out the old as you open yourself up to novel and inspirational ideas.

## IN WITH THE NEW

After the glaciers retreated at the end of the last ice age, the birch trees were the first to colonize and heal that icy, excoriated land. They gave of themselves to nourish the soil. Referred to as a pioneer tree, birch matures quickly, then dies and breaks down, enriching the soil so that other, longer-living noble trees like oak and beech can grow and form old forests, and habitats for birds and animals. It is because of this that the birch is seen as the tree of new beginnings, fresh starts. She sweeps away the old and heralds in the new, but she gives of herself for the greater good of the whole community.

# DETOXIFICATION AND BIOPHOTONS

Life is so different now. It is difficult for us to remember that not long ago, the food you grew on your small farm, or foraged from the land around you, was the food you ate. When that ran out, you starved. By the time they had made it to the Spring Equinox, our ancestors were lucky if they still had some food left over in their stores. This period was known as the hunger gap, when the last year's stores were very low but new food was scarce on the ground.

After a hard winter, the people admired the re-youthing of the herbage and trees surrounding their homes with their bright green foliage and energetic growth spurt. Seeking to acquire some of that energy, they did so by eating the fresh green shoots. The medieval pottage is a cauldron of grains, greens, mushrooms, and some bones or meat if you were lucky. Along with bread and ale, this was the mainstay of their diet, and their source of vitamins and minerals came from the fresh green herbs around them – the same herbs we call weeds.

After spending winter nestled under a blanket of composting leaves, the roots reach down into the soil of Mother Earth, drawing minerals upwards. The leaves stretch upward, drawing sunlight down into the plant where, under the guidance of nature, the two sources of nourishment combine, as if in an alchemist's crucible, to produce the specific combination of that plant's biochemical profile, which provides not only food but also medicine for both two- and four-legged animals. Both fell with relish upon the abundance of greenery, and profited from that alchemical substance within those green cells.

Today, we live in a toxic world. Fortunately, we are slowly waking up, and using our people-power to demand that the greener solutions, which are well known to technology and that can sustainably provide food and energy, be put into place by our governments. With hope, we can preserve the exquisite beauty and diversity of this magnificent blue orb upon which we have the enormous privilege to spend our lives. For now, let us turn our attention to detoxifying our own bodies using the herbage of springtime, for nature is ever generous, providing us with detoxification medicines from the very plants that so many choose to poison, because they call them weeds. We call them awesome!

◢ ◢ ◢

Hippocrates instructed us to "Let food be thy medicine and medicine be thy food", and I do think that, like our ancestors, we have a natural urge to eat cleansing foods in the springtime. The taste of wild herbage can be challenging to get your lips around, but once included in innovative recipes, they become meals to look forward to and relish every spring. Of course, it brings us back to nature again, to live in tune with the seasons. So, let us begin with the most famous of all wild food, the noble nettle, beloved of naughty school boys, and folks with weird fetishes.

## Nettle (*Urtica dioica*)

Nettles are rich in protein, vitamin A, silica, calcium and iron, which makes this a wonderful herb, especially for women of all ages, as it tops up our natural mineral levels. Men, of course, also benefit, but they don't tend to lose bone density or iron as much as women do. The vitamin A stimulates hair growth and reduces the tendency toward acne, calcium supports bone density, and iron and protein support hair growth and supplement the iron lost through menstruation. The herb also contains selenium, zinc and some magnesium, as well as vitamin C and B vitamins, so within this humble weed lies a veritable multivitamin and mineral complex.

Herbalists have always used nettles to cleanse the body, and we find this herb particularly helpful for sufferers of eczema, arthritis and gout. Traditionally, we say that nettles clear uric acid crystals and inflammatory materials out of the blood via the kidneys. It is my experience that my patients benefit enormously when nettle is included in their herbal prescriptions.

Whenever I am asked to help someone with hair loss, nettles always feature in the prescription, and after only a few weeks, I have a delighted patient requesting more of the prescription. I do remember one lady who had recently had an operation on her intestine, and her hair had started falling out in chunks. I reasoned that the inflammation in her intestine prior to and after the operation had probably inhibited her absorption of nutrients, and gave her a tonic with a hefty dose of nettles. Within a few weeks she happily reported that she now looked like a pineapple with thick spikes of new hair growth all over her head. But then she went on to exclaim, "But what it's done for my hands!" She is a piano player, and she hadn't told me that her hands were becoming stiff and sore with the onset of arthritis. The nettles had given her her hands and hair back, and she became a nettle devotee.

Herbalists have found that when people develop acne spots, it can be the result of toxins, and the body trying to flush them out via the largest organ of elimination in our bodies: the skin. This may be because the major organs of detoxification are working under par, and thus it makes sense to support the kidneys and liver when doing any detox programme. For skin conditions, we find that using herbs to help the body to be rid of toxins can really help to clear the complexion, when taken over a period of time. Although nettles work via the kidneys and the liver, I like to support all the organs of elimination when I am doing a detox, so you will find a detox recipe at the end of the chapter.

I know that as a herbalist, I am supposed to love nettle soup. But I don't. I find it a bit green in flavour. However, mixed with wild garlic, it becomes utterly sublime. You need to collect the nettles when they are very young, otherwise you will have stringy soup – yuk. It is fun picking nettles, and don't worry too much about the stings – they are good for you.

## NETTLE AND WILD GARLIC SOUP

🌿 Start with a good stock, as described on page 13. Warm it gently.

🌿 Snip the tops of young nettles. Collect some wild garlic at the same time.

🌿 Pick the leaves off the nettle stems, so that you have a good handful of leaves – rinse them off and dry on a cloth.

🌿 Rinse 1 or even 2 handfuls of wild garlic and dry on a cloth.

🌿 Now add to your stock a few scrubbed potatoes which have been cubed, and cook them in the stock until they are soft. If you eat meat, you might like to throw in a rasher or two of smoked bacon for extra flavour.

🌿 Now that the potatoes are soft, toss in your leaves and stir. They will quickly collapse into the hot liquid. Allow them 5 minutes to cook and soften. Now retrieve your bacon and give it to your dog or local fox, and allow the soup to cool a little before pureeing in your food processor until very smooth. Grind in some sea salt and black pepper.

🌿 Swirl in a little double (heavy) cream. Serve with crusty bread and good fresh butter.

🌿 This soup is absolutely luscious.

*It is fun picking nettles, and don't worry too much about the stings – they are good for you.*

## Ground elder (*Aegopodium podagraria*)

The English gardener and herbalist John Gerard (1545–1611) rather famously complained bitterly about this plant being "so fruitful in his increase, that where once it hath taken root, it will hardly be gotten out again, spoiling and getting every yeere more ground, to the annoying of better herbes" – and no doubt to the annoying of all gardeners ever since.

The Romans brought it to Britain as a pot herb, and indeed, it is quite nice when steamed and drizzled with butter in the springtime, rather like asparagus. In fact, the two complement each other nicely as they are both cleansing diuretics. Alternatively, enjoy its refreshing lemony taste as a tea.

Ground elder has an affinity for the urinary system, and as such can be seen as a cleansing, detoxifying and slimming herb. When combined with a cleansing, reduced-calorie diet, the diuretic herbs do contribute toward a more svelte figure. But this most unloved herb gives us more. It is able to produce so much vitamin C that it was once used to treat scurvy.

We shall come back to ground elder in a later chapter when we look at arthritis and gout, but for now, do remember that vitamin C is an essential building block for collagen, and therefore prolonging your youthful complexion. Cleansing the toxins out of our bodies leaves us with fresher, brighter skin, eyes and hair, with a much more supple body. The removal of excess fluids helps to keep us slim and the enhanced vitamin and mineral content of these weeds brings obvious health benefits. For what is it that makes us physically beautiful, but the skin, hair and figure of a vibrantly healthy person? Your beauty comes from the health within your body.

Your health also comes from the food that you eat, and our wild weeds provide superb spring vegetables. Do give ground elder a chance. The young leaves have an almost transparent, radiant lime-green colour, and a fresh lemony taste. Indeed, they do make an interesting addition to our vegetable table.

## GROUND ELDER, NETTLE AND WILD GARLIC RISOTTO

Gather a handful of young ground elder leaves, nettle tops and wild garlic leaves.

Wash, pat dry and chop roughly.

Sautee an onion, and add risotto rice to the pan, coating the rice in the oil.

Slowly add a good chicken or vegetable stock, stirring as the rice absorbs the liquid.

When the rice has softened and absorbed all the liquid, add the herbs and allow to thoroughly wilt.

Serve with a sprinkle of dandelion and chive petals and some Parmesan cheese.

## ASPARAGUS WITH GROUND ELDER

Steam a bunch of asparagus.

Drizzle with butter or olive oil.

Garnish with a generous sprinkle of finely chopped young ground elder leaves.

To make this a meal in itself, crumble tangy feta over the top. Serve with a tomato salad, crusty French bread and olive oil.

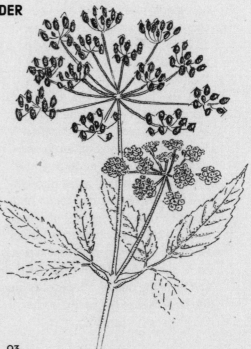

## Burdock (*Arctium lappa*)

Burdock is the don of the hedgerow. It's big, handsome and packs a powerful punch when it comes to cleansing out the rubbish stored in our cells. The root has liver-protecting qualities due to its powerful antioxidant actions, and as such, it clears up the free-radical louts which damage your cells. The root also has diuretic actions, thus washing the toxins out of the body. Medical herbalists use burdock root as a deep cleanse, to remove the toxins packed away in your cells. This can be tricky because the body needs to be carefully prepared in order to be able to remove these toxins quickly and safely out of the body. If the body is not correctly prepared, a healing crisis can occur where the person breaks out in eczema, or suffers from headaches, fatigue and nausea – much like a hangover.

Detoxification of the cells needs the support of all the organs of elimination. Burdock is our hefty tough guy who releases the toxins and takes them out of the body, but he needs allies. I like to use a circulatory stimulant like ginger to help to flush the cells with fresh blood. The blood will carry the toxins out of the tissues into the blood vessels, to the kidneys and the liver where they are "processed" for elimination. The diuretic actions of nettle and dandelion leaves encourage the toxins to be washed away through the kidneys, whilst dandelion and burdock roots encourage the liver to flush the toxins into the bowel. Finally, I like to include chia, flaxseeds and dock root (*Rumex crispus*) to stimulate the bowel, effectively slipping the toxic faeces out of the body.

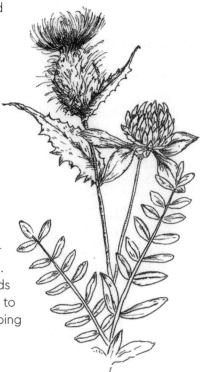

By opening up the channels of elimination, the body is not forced to eliminate via the skin, and soon you should find that you have lovely clear skin. However, acne is also caused by bacteria, which live on your skin, feeding off the oils in your sebum. This is why antibiotics work so well, but they do have detrimental effects on the body. Burdock root and leaves have natural antibacterial actions, in particular against the bacteria which cause acne.

The seeds have a role to play as well. Seeds hold the fats of the plant. Burdock seeds seem to have a balancing effect on the sebum secretion of our skin, and may be particularly helpful for dry, itchy conditions such as eczema. Look at the burrs of burdock. They are the prickly things which hold the seeds. If you got some burrs stuck inside your clothing, they would irritate your skin and make you scratch. In this way, they are almost telling you why you would want to use them.

Burdock has also been found to be helpful for cystitis – another burning, irritating condition. The roots are not only antibacterial, but they disrupt the biofilm layer. Bacteria are clever; they don't want to be killed by antibiotics, so they live in communities within a slimy biofilm layer, which shelters the bacteria from antibiotics. Burdock disrupts this layer, making the bacteria vulnerable to the herb's natural antibacterial action, as well as other herbal antibacterials.[29] [30]

I love burdock. I love to stand next to the plant in the hedgerow and stroke their big rough leaves. They remind me of elephant's ears.

## Clivers (*Galium aparine*)

Herbalists value clivers for its effect on the watery systems of our bodies. This herb cleanses the lymphatic system, and is especially useful in the treatment of swollen glands caused by bacterial or viral infection.

In the past, a bunch of clivers was bundled up and used as a sieve to separate curds from whey, and this image gives us a good idea of how the herb works within the lymphatic system. Dead bacteria, old cells and other debris are captured in the sieve-like apparatus of the lymph nodes, which can become congested and swollen. Clivers helps to decongest the lymphatic system, by washing the debris out of the lymph, into the kidneys and out of the body. Do be careful here, because glands swell for reasons, and if they don't return to their normal size within a week, you must see your doctor. Having said that, for those who have had tonsilitis, or following glandular fever, this herb is a safe and refreshing tonic to the lymph glands.

There is an old saying: "Drink clivers to be slim and svelte like the herb." It has a reputation for alleviating cellulite, but perhaps more realistically, it gently shifts the stagnant fluid in the tissues, so that you shrink a little.

As an aside, when my patients ask me to provide for them a slimming diet, I start a little light-heartedly by suggesting that they look at the shape of their food. For instance, if you want to look like a potato, then eat potatoes. If you want to be puffed up like a croissant, then eat croissants. If you want to be slim and lean like a leek or asparagus, then eat leeks and asparagus.

## SLIMMER'S TEA

🌿 Pull a handful of clivers from the hedge and roll it into a ball.

🌿 Collect 4 dandelion leaves and drop into a cup of boiling water, then add your clivers.

🌿 Allow to steep for an hour, then strain.

🌿 Add the juice of half a grapefruit and drink.

## DETOXING PROTOCOL

**PHASE 1:** During this phase, we use herbs to cleanse and decongest the major organs of elimination, so that when the toxins are released from the cells, they can be quickly eliminated from the body. For now, we focus on the kidneys, liver and bowels.

**FOLLOW THIS FOR 2 WEEKS:**

1 tsp freshly chopped celery leaves
  (kidney support)
1 tsp freshly grated ginger root
  (liver support)
½ tsp freshly grated turmeric root
  (liver support)
2 tsp roughly chopped clivers
  (kidney and lymphatic support)
1 tsp finely chopped birch leaves
  (kidney support – avoid if allergic
  to aspirin)
juice from ½ a freshly squeezed lemon
  (liver support)
chia seeds

🌿 Of this herbal mixture, take 2 teaspoons daily. The rest can be refrigerated for the next few days.

🌿 In the evening, pour 2 cups of boiling water over the herbs and allow to steep for 20 minutes. Strain, and pour into two separate glasses, then stir into each glass 1 teaspoon of chia seeds. Leave overnight. In the morning, drink 1 cup of this gloopy infusion, and again in the evening.

🌿 Include in your diet plenty of celery, grapefruit, vegetables, pulses, vegetable soups, salads, fruit, nuts and seeds, and some rice. Radically reduce or avoid meats, and completely avoid wheat, dairy and sugar. Drink plenty of water or herbal teas throughout the day.

**Phase 2:** During this phase, we continue to support the organs of elimination, but we go deeper into the cells. You might find it easier to purchase some of the herbs, as digging up a burdock root is sometimes unrealistic for people living in town. Continue following the dietary suggestions on page 97.

**FOLLOW THIS FOR 2 WEEKS:**

1 tsp fresh or ½ tsp dried dandelion root (liver support)

1 tsp finely chopped fresh dandelion leaf (kidney support)

1 tsp finely chopped celery leaf (kidney support)

1 tsp fresh burdock leaf (cellular cleansing)

¼ tsp dried burdock root (cellular cleansing)

1 tsp freshly grated ginger root (circulatory stimulant, liver support)

1 tsp finely chopped parsley leaves (kidney support – do not use if pregnant)

chia seeds

🌿 Of this mixture of herbs, take 2 teaspoons and add to a teapot with 2 cups of boiling water. The rest can be placed in an airproof container and kept in the refrigerator for the next day.

🌿 Allow to steep for 30 minutes, then strain. Divide into two glasses and add 1 teaspoon of chia seeds to each. Stir and leave overnight. In the morning, drink 1 glass before food, and again in the evening.

🌿 It helps the detoxification process if you include a programme of intermittent fasting, which allows the body to focus on clearing out the toxins without having to deal with digesting and absorbing foods. To do this, you can restrict eating times to 6 hours a day, leaving your body 18 hours to cleanse. The usual hours are that you eat from noon until 6pm, then nothing except herbal teas until noon again. As a concession, a cup of tea or coffee in the morning will make life so much more bearable for most people.

## Chickweed (*Stellaria media)*

Traditionally, herbalists love to use chickweed for skin conditions such as eczema, or for the "inner skin", the mucous membrane of the gut, in cases such as gastritis. But before I tell you more about that, I want to enlarge upon chickweed, because this interesting little plant does have more to offer.

Chickweed is so named because it is fed to chickens, who love its soft leaves, rich in nutrients. Whilst it fattens chickens, it actually has a slimming effect on us, which it achieves through at least two mechanisms. First, the natural chemical β-sitosterol competes with dietary fat and reduces fat absorption, and secondly it restrains the digestive enzymes lipase and amylase, which break the fat down and facilitate its absorption.[31]

For such a weedy little plant, it is actually quite punchy, and has been discovered to have potent anti-hepatitis B viral activity.[32]

Being particularly rich in calcium, it may be useful for defending against the onset of osteoporosis as an alternative source of calcium to dairy. These effects are best achieved when turning chickweed into a juice, so do include a handful in your smoothie or juice. It is also healing for those suffering from gastritis, and in this case a chopped tablespoon or two daily should be sufficient. If you don't want to juice, then simply add this to your salads or top your pasta. Chickweed can even be turned into a pesto.

The plant is very soft and cool, and these are the properties that we seek to harness when we prescribe the herb for inflamed conditions of the skin or inner membranes of the body. To illustrate the point: imagine a hot summer's day, when your face is burning from the heat. You lay your hot face against a cool mound of chickweed, and the heat is absorbed by the plant, leaving soft, soothed skin. Chickweed is a wonderful herb to use for eczema of the skin, and is very safe.

I love to walk the lonely paths in the hills surrounding my village home. High up, under the oaks, roam the cows, who fertilize the soil, and upon that fertile soil grows luscious patches of chickweed. It is often found growing on compost heaps too.

## COOLING CHICKWEED GEL FOR ECZEMA

I suggest making this gel with aloe vera gel, because aloe is rich in allantoin, a natural compound found in many plants, especially aloe and comfrey leaves. Allantoin holds water in the cells and strengthens the matrix beneath the skin, in this way giving us a more youthful, dewy appearance. It is the perfect accompaniment to chickweed for irritated skin, but this gel would also be wonderful to help keep skin youthful.

🌿 Harvest a handful or two of chickweed, and bring it home, rinse it off and pat dry. Leave overnight, then place it in a small saucepan and pour about 200ml (7fl oz) of almond oil over the plant matter. Place the saucepan into a frying pan of simmering water, creating a bain-marie.

🌿 If you can find some fresh German chamomile or calendula flowers, do add these to your chickweed, because they have fantastic anti-inflammatory and healing properties.

🌿 As the oil warms, it will extract the healing constituents from the herbs. Allow the extraction to continue for about an hour, then switch off the heat, but leave the pans in place to slowly cool.

🌿 Strain the herbs from the oil through muslin into a glass bottle and add 20 drops of geranium essential oil to preserve. Keep in the refrigerator.

🌿 To make your gel, purchase a tube or pot of good-quality aloe vera gel. Make sure that you do not use a gel which is made from whole leaf extract. You only want the filleted inner leaf extract.

🌿 Whisk 10–15ml (2–3 teaspoons) of chickweed oil into 45ml (3 tablespoons) of aloe vera gel, so that you now have an opaque gel.

🌿 You might want to add a total of 10 drops of essential oils such as frankincense, lavender or carrot seed oil, all of which are valued for their skin-healing qualities.

🌿 This will give you 60ml (2fl oz) of gel to apply to hot itchy eczema.

🌿 **CAUTION:** Do not use calendula or chamomile if you are allergic to the daisy family.

# Horsetail (*Equisetum arvense*)

Along with nettles, horsetail is another plague of the gardener. If only the gardener understood that rather than tossing away handfuls of the weeds, she could be drinking an infusion of horsetail and nettles, and in so doing, growing abundant hair and strong nails, as well as toning her varicose veins – for both are rich in silica, which fortifies collagen, the matrix which gives strength to our tissues.

Medical herbalists use this herb for all conditions related to weak collagen. The silica is water soluble and readily available to the body to use as a mineral. We use horsetail to strengthen breaking nails, weak veins such as varicose veins and piles, weak hair, weak bladders and weak lungs, and it is sometimes helpful for prolapses. Leg ulcers, which are slow to heal, can also be helped with a poultice of pulverized horsetail herb and honey. When I say "weak", I refer to the tone of the organ wall which has become weakened and therefore less able to hold urine, blood or work effectively in the case of the lungs. Horsetail strengthens the matrix of the organ wall.

To grow strong, luscious locks, you need a good flow of blood to the scalp, which will deliver nutrients to the hair follicle. Rosemary improves blood flow to the head and it is a traditional hair tonic, but also remember your one hundred brush strokes a day. Iron and silica produce good-quality hair. The three herbs in your garden which can provide these actions are rosemary, nettles and horsetail. This combination can be used as a final rinse to strengthen the hair shafts.

**CAUTION:** Please do not use rosemary if you have a tendency toward or have ever had a seizure.

## STRENGTHENING HAIR RINSE

This hair rinse not only strengthens the hair shaft, but as the herbs soak into the scalp, they encourage the fresh growth of new, strong hair. The apple cider vinegar lowers the pH to a healthier acidity, which strengthens and smooths the hair, giving it a healthy, glossy appearance.

1 handful of fresh or dried
    nettle tops
1 handful of fresh or dried
    horsetail tops
a generous sprig of rosemary, or
    2 drops of rosemary essential oil
2 tbsp apple cider vinegar

Pour boiling water over the nettles, horsetail herb and rosemary, quickly cover with a lid, and allow to infuse all day.

Strain the herbs out, reserving the precious liquid. If you haven't used rosemary herb, you can add the essential oil at this point.

Add the apple cider vinegar, and you might like to gently reheat so that you don't feel too much of a cold shock as you pour this over your hair as a final rinse. Do not rinse out, just squeeze dry and then dry as usual.

*This hair rinse not only strengthens the hair shaft, but as the herbs soak into the scalp, they encourage the fresh growth of new, strong hair.*

# BIOPHOTONS - THE LIGHT OF LIFE

You are a light in the dark. Every time the DNA in our cells contracts, an information-encoded particle of light called a biophoton is emitted. Each of these communicates the DNA information from that individual cell to other biophotons, both inside the body and also to the biophoton field surrounding the body. Thus, our body's cells are all connected by a dynamic web of light that is constantly being released and absorbed by our DNA.

All living organisms (humans, plants and animals) are bathed in this inner light generated from our cellular DNA. These extremely weak and invisible particles of light called biophotons were first discovered by Alexander Gurwitsch in the 1920s, for which he received the Stalin Prize for his work.

Biophotons seem to be the vehicle by which all our metabolic information is carried around our bodies. This information-carrying biophoton light regulates the activity of all our life processes. It has a highly coherent vibration, and the vibrational information literally moves at the speed of light.

The light not only bathes our cells, but creates a biophoton field (an invisible light field of information) around our bodies, which allows us to interact with the biophoton fields of other bodies. This is a possible explanation as to how flocks of birds or schools of fish are able to move collectively, so instantly and cohesively. Perhaps it also explains how people who share a close relationship have the same ideas at the same time.

It is the high level of vibrational coherence that these information-carrying biophotons confer which is so important to our health. In the 1970s, Dr Fritz-Albert Popp proposed that good health is "a state of perfect subatomic coherent communication, and ill health is a state of communication breakdown".

Popp also found that carcinogenic chemicals can be recognized by their property of disrupting biophoton emissions and the coherence of light waves. He found that when the natural cycles of our light emissions are disrupted, the light waves lose their coherence, and illnesses such as cancer ensue.

Based on this, he surmised that there must be compounds which have the effect of restoring coherence to the biophoton emissions, and health. When he tested mistletoe, he found that the herb was able to return the disrupted biophoton emissions of cancer cells back to normal, and the cancer went into remission.

Popp went on to discover that the healthiest food had the most coherent emissions of light, and that biophotons can be transmitted to us from plants.[33] [34] The biophotons derived from our plant food are able to restore order, and in that way, restore our health.

Measurements of biophotons in food have led to an amazing discovery. The foods richest in biophotons – thus having the ability to bring coherent, healing vibrational information into our bodies – are wild plants such as berries, nettles and dandelions.

We know that medical plants are made up of hundreds of natural constituents which can have a beneficial or toxic effect on our bodies, but that is a biochemical mechanism. Biophotons offer a different mechanism, for it is the vibrational information signature of light from the biophotons which the herbs are transmitting to us. Herbs have affinities for certain parts of our bodies, for instance hawthorn supports the heart, while elecampane supports the lungs. Perhaps the biophotons from these herbs hold a vibrational signature, like a blueprint, which perfectly matches the cellular vibrational signature of healthy tissue cells in those body systems. Thus when we ingest the plant as medicine, they are able to transfer that coherent biophoton signature to our cells, thereby restoring the correct information for cellular health.

But how, dear reader, can you use this information in your everyday life? Young nettle tops, tender dandelion and ground elder leaves, wild garlic and the berries of the late summer are all pulsing with the vibrant and coherent biophoton life force. Pick them and eat them within two hours of harvest so that you capture within your cells the light of vibrant health. Biophotons have been shown to inhibit entropy (ageing and decay); they literally bring life and health back to us – so do eat them in as great quantities as you can manage. Flood your body with green light.

Biophoton study goes further. It has been discovered only recently that our own "mental intentions" can influence these biophoton emissions, both within our own bodies and others, even at a great distance. A 2012 study found that when subjects placed in a very dark environment were asked to simply imagine light, their intention alone produced significant increases in biophoton emissions from their heads.[35]

The mechanism by which intention works seems to be by magnifying an electromagnetic energy field which produces an orderly discharge of biophotons. These highly coherent frequencies, generated as a result of human intention, can change the structure of matter, even at a distance.

It seems that it is the intention which generates the biophotons and charges the electromagnetic fields, which may be the mechanism by which extremely ill people suddenly go into remission, whether the healer is present or not. The biophotons deliver coherent healing information to the cells at the speed of light. I should be clear that people can also heal themselves through intention, or through prayer.

Every living being on this planet emits biophoton information. We are all so much more than merely a collection of mechanistic atoms and molecules. Rather, we are truly beings who emit, communicate through, and are actually formed from light. We are beings of light, healed by the light of plants, and able to send each other "love and light". Plants and humans – we simply are light itself.

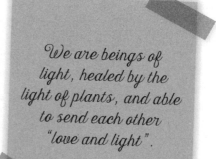

*We are beings of light, healed by the light of plants, and able to send each other "love and light".*

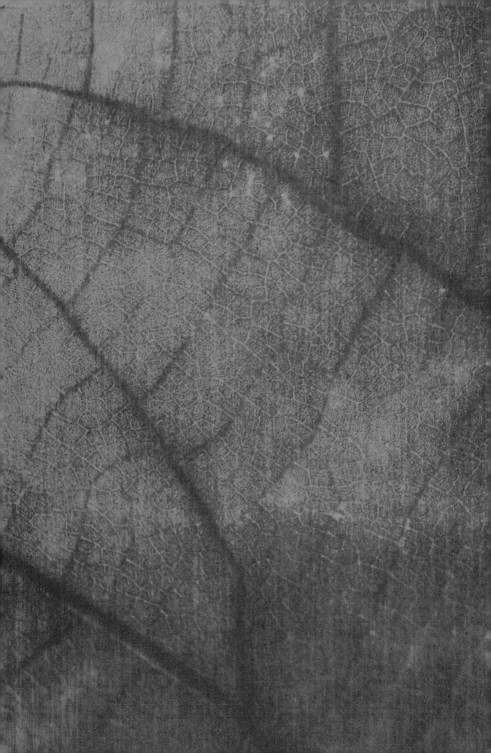

# CHAPTER 4

## Beltane and the Fields of Your Heart

'Tis the merry month of May, and the flowers are unfurling their petals, flirting with the bees who fertilize them, and bringing an abundance of honey and fruit to the land. We cannot help noticing the hawthorn tree in bloom everywhere. Indeed, the whole countryside is festooned with the dainty bridal lacework of this tree. Also known as May blossom, she is a tree of the heart, of love and joy, and the queen of the Celtic festival of Beltane, which celebrates the fertility of the land. This ancient fire ceremony is one of the most joyous Celtic festivals of the year.

On the morning of Beltane eve, for hundreds of years, local people go 'a-Maying', collecting boughs of May blossom which will adorn the bride of woodlands – the Goddess. On this day, the Lord and Lady of the Woods join together in love and a festival of fertility, to bless the land with rich crops. To this effect, a maiden from the community is selected to represent the Goddess. She is dressed in boughs of May blossom, and processed to meet a young man representing the Lord of the Wood. Everyone joins in, and there is merriment and dancing around the maypole.

It is said that in the past, on Beltane eve, as far as the eye could see, every hilltop was ablaze with the Beltane fires, around which crowds gathered to dance, jump the fires, and ask for the blessings of the God and the Goddess. Everyone was there, even the sheep and cattle who were driven through the smoke to rid them of the fleas and ticks. The Earth was heady with mead, laughter and love, and love brings new life. The babies conceived that night were known as merry-begots.

In the morning, the coals from the Beltane fires were used to relight the hearths of every home, and a handful of ash was scattered upon every field, so that the whole of the land, and all who live upon her, were blessed with the love of the God and the Goddess, that the cycle of life may continue.

Hawthorn is the tree of the heart, on every level. In the southwest of England there is a rich legend that Joseph of Arimathea brought the message of spiritual love from Jesus to this land. He arrived carrying a staff, which when struck into the earth at Glastonbury, sprouted leaves and became the famous Glastonbury Thorn. A sprig from a scion of this tree is sent to the Queen's Christmas table each year, and I know this because I have met the man who used to perform this annual ritual.

For the emotional heart, I like to use the petals of hawthorn flowers, combined with roses and linden blossom, to soothe a broken heart. The leaves and fruits I keep for conditions of the physical heart.

This tree is not all about rosy petals. There are thorns and she is bent and twisted by the winds of life, but like true love, she endures. The Druids call her Huathe. To them too, this is a tree of the heart and courage. To me, this is a tree which grows in wild places. Not so much a pretty garden tree as a wildly beautiful hag. In Cornwall, for instance, you will find very few trees which grow on that windy peninsula, but there she is, our beautiful Huathe. The winds of life have bent her to almost 45 degrees, and yet she endures. In my heart, I can hear her screaming with ecstatic joy into the battering winds. It feels to me as if she revels in her loneliness and wildness, yet she welcomes the wayfarer who shelters under her branches. She grows where she will. She is not tamed by the pruning of garden clippers. No, this tree follows her own direction and that of the winds.

## THE FIELDS OF OUR HEART

Our planet is cushioned within a powerful protective electromagnetic field, which is generated from the iron-rich heart of the Earth, 3,000km beneath our feet. We, too, generate an electromagnetic field from our brains, but also from our hearts – the electric field of our heart is 100 times stronger than that of our brain, and the heart's magnetic field is 5,000 times stronger than the brain's. Our physical body, like the Earth, is cushioned within fields of energy, directed not by our brains but by our hearts. These fields have a lot of power.

Within our hearts is a collection of neurons which scientists call "the little brain of the heart". But it is not so little, because they discovered that more messages are transmitted toward the brain from the heart than the other way around. We are heart-intelligent beings. Why does this matter? Because how we feel within our hearts affects our planetary consciousness.

You can think of each one of us as a single neuron within the brain of the whole (the whole being our planet, or indeed the universe, for that matter). Collectively, if the neurons choose to express co-operation, the organism benefits. If each thinks only for itself, the organism ultimately dies – like cancer. This knowledge gives each one of us the power to change the world for the better. It is known as subtle activism.

On 6 September 2011, the National Geographic Society Newsroom reported on what is known as the Global Consciousness Project, which uses a programme dubbed "EGG", meaning electrogaiagram, because its design is reminiscent of an EEG (electric encephalogram) for the Earth. The project uses high technology to explore whether there is any evidence of communal global consciousness. The electromagnetic fields of the Earth follow a fairly predictable vibrational pattern, but at the time of the 9/11 attacks, and for five hours afterward, they noted a sharp and significant spike in the electromagnetic fields. The scientists said, "The network responded as if the coherence and intensity of our common reaction created a sustained pulse of order in the random flow of numbers from our instruments. These patterns where there should be none, look like reflections of our concentrated focus of attention, as the riveting events drew us from our individual concerns and melded us into an extraordinary shared state. Maybe we became, briefly, a coherent global consciousness."[36]

The paper refers to our emotional response, which is generated from the powerful electromagnetic fields of our hearts. From this we may wonder: what effect would our combined consciousness have if each of us were to make sustained efforts to generate from our heart a feeling of love and healing toward all beings of the world? We have the potential to be magnificent co-creators, and it all comes from our hearts.

The Maharishi Effect refers to over 50 studies conducted by the Maharishi Vedic Research Institute on the effect of sustained meditative individual consciousness of a group, on society as a whole. Individual consciousness, as determined by the quality of thoughts and behaviour, is a unit within the collective consciousness which influences, or may be influenced by, the collective group consciousness.

They believe that events such as acts of terrorism or war are a bursting-out of the group consciousness of a stressful society, and that by maintaining a coherent and simultaneous group consciousness of peace and love, we can change the world. Their studies have shown that when groups practise meditation or yoga techniques, there are significant reductions in crime, accidents, mortality, war and terrorism, and improvements in economic indicators and the general quality of life. They have also predicted that a meditation group, equal to the size of the square root of one per cent of a population, would have a measurable beneficial influence on the quality of life of that population.[37]

Knowing that the energy frequency generated from the thoughts in our brains and the feelings from our hearts carries so much potential to contribute toward a better world, let us now turn back toward the herbs which support our heart, because it seems the strength of our heart is important not just to ourselves, but possibly for the enhancement of our planetary consciousness, and the very survival of most species sharing this planet with us.

*Let us now turn back toward the herbs which support our heart, because it seems the strength of our heart is important not just to ourselves, but possibly for the enhancement of our planetary consciousness.*

# HERBS FOR THE HEART

🌿 HAWTHORN 🌿 SLOES 🌿 LINDEN BLOSSOM
🌿 YARROW 🌿 DANDELION LEAF 🌿 MOTHERWORT
🌿 OLIVE LEAF 🌿 HORSE CHESTNUT 🌿 OAK LEAVES

In 2017, according to the World Health Organization, 9.4 million people died of heart disease, and 5.8 million died of strokes. With herbal medicine and a decent diet, there is a lot that can be done to keep our hearts and the blood vessels in good health, and assuage the effects of the modern Western lifestyle which is so much the underlying cause of these figures.

Within the vegetable world is a large group of phytonutrients called flavonoids. This class of nutrients can be divided into subgroups, but the take-home message is that these colourful nutrients are extremely beneficial for the heart, the blood vessels and of course, the rest of our body. Simply being alive means that we are experiencing oxidative damage to our cells all the time, which leads to a wide range of diseases; cardiac disease, age-related dementia and cancers being the big ones. The good news is that the flavonoids are the antidote, as they are antioxidant in action. This means that we are able to hugely offset the negative effects of oxidation through our dietary choices, although we must also accept that ageing comes to us all. But we can age in good style.

We all know this by now, but I am going to say it again: deep-fat-fried, highly processed, sugary and low-fibre foods are all extremely damaging to our health. Your fish and chips are fine as a treat, once, when you are on holiday at the seaside, but when it happens every Friday night, then you develop bad habits which are difficult to break and hard on your heart.

# A DIET FOR A HEALTHY HEART

The brilliant news is that some of our most beloved treats are naturally high in antioxidants, so do enjoy your chocolate (only very dark please), tea, coffee and red wine. When I am consulting, I always notice a wheeze of relief escaping the lips of my patients as they joyfully absorb this nugget of news.

Flavonoids are colourful, which is why the rainbow diet is so healthy. Your rule of thumb is to look for colourful foods and eat as much of these as you can.

## Healthy fats

You also need to include healthy fats in your diet, with a nice spectrum of omega-3, -6, -7 and -9.

### Omega-3

Foods rich in omega-3 have an anti-inflammatory effect and help to protect the blood vessels, reduce the build-up of plaques in the blood vessel walls, regulate the heartbeat and help to prevent blood clots.

### Omega-6

Omega-6 fats receive a bad rap, but recent evidence suggests the fatty acid DGLA (dihomo-gamma-linolenic acid) can actually help to stop the hardening of the arteries so intricately associated with cardiac disease. GLA, from which DGLA is derived, is not found in many foodstuffs, but it is present in evening primrose oil, hemp, blackcurrant and borage seed oils, and spirulina.

### Omega-7

Unlike omegas-3 and -6, omega-7s are classed as non-essential fatty acids because our bodies can make these ourselves. One of the most common omega-7s has recently received attention because it acts like a hormone. This fatty acid, known as palmitoleic acid, is produced by our own fat and liver cells, but travels to our blood vessels where it enhances insulin sensitivity of the cells, thus helping to prevent the onset of metabolic syndrome or diabetes. It helps to correct cholesterol levels, and may reduce the incidence of heart attacks.[38]

**Omega-9**

Omega-9 fatty acids are also classed as non-essential, because our body can manufacture them endogenously. They offer health benefits such as balancing our cholesterol profile and helping to protect against age-related dementia.

**Foods rich in flavonoids include:**

- Dark-skinned berries, such as blueberries, raspberries, red and black grapes and blackberries

- Orange vegetables, such as sweet potato, butternut squash and carrots

- Red and purple vegetables, such as beetroot (beets), tomatoes, red (bell) peppers, aubergine (eggplant) and red cabbage

- Green vegetables, such as kale, lettuce, leek and spinach

- Lentils, kidney beans and black beans

**Foods rich in omega-3 include:**

- Walnuts, flaxseeds, pumpkin seeds, hemp seeds and chia

- Seaweeds and algae

- Oily fish such as mackerel, herring, pilchards, sardines, salmon and trout

**Foods rich in omega-6 include:**

- Sunflower seeds, almonds, cashews, hemp seeds

- Avocado, pear

- Eggs (free-range organic please)

**Foods rich in omega-7 include:**

- Sea buckthorn (not easily accessible)
- Avocados
- Olive oil
- Raw macadamia nuts

**Foods rich in omega-9 include:**

- Olive oil
- Sunflower seeds
- Almonds
- Avocados

**Other foods which are particularly helpful for the cardiac and circulatory system include:**

- Garlic and onions
- Hummus
- Beetroot (beets)
- Olives and olive oil
- Salad leaves
- Fresh herbs
- Tomatoes
- Lemons and limes
- Porridge oats
- Ginger

Try to base your diet on a high proportion of colourful vegetables, salads and fruits, with some heathy nuts and seeds, and two to three portions of oily fish a week. This is not to say that you cannot enjoy some red meat or chicken, or roast potatoes – just tip the balance toward the foods listed above. Now, to the herbs ...

## Hawthorn (*Crataegus spp.*)

Hawthorn is THE tree for the heart. It is a very safe option for its action is slow but sure. This is my number one herb for cardiac failure, and is indicated for low to moderate heart failure, although I have used it for severe heart failure too. Hawthorn is not a bells and whistles herb, so the person may not notice massive changes, and yet, hawthorn gently keeps the heart going for years longer than might have been anticipated. This is not a herb to forego if you have a weak heart, because this herb will give your heart strength.

The flowers, leaves, seeds and berries all contribute to the herb's healing properties. I like to collect the flowers and leaves in May, and the berries in September, then blend all parts of the plant together in one tincture for a well-rounded therapeutic effect.

The action for which hawthorn is so famous is its ability to dilate the coronary blood vessels. It is thought to do this by nitric oxide, the same chemical used in Viagra, but of course, much milder. By opening the blood vessels supplying the cardiac muscle, nutrients are delivered into the muscle, giving it strength and nourishment. Your heart has been beating on average 70 times a minute since you were six weeks old in your mother's womb. After several decades of climbing mountains, smoking or air pollution, stress, falling in and out of love – it can feel weary. It needs a little kindness and some extra nourishment. This is where hawthorn comes in – we call it the Mother of the Old Heart.

The berries and leaves are rich in bioflavonoids. Flavonoids not only mop up free radicals, but they reduce inflammation and strengthen the walls of the blood vessels. In this way they protect against blood clots and strokes. When the blood vessel is damaged, the platelets in the bloodstream start to clump together, and adhere to the wall of the blood vessel in order to heal its damaged lining. Long strands of fibrin entangle with the platelets and a blood clot is formed. If the clot dislodges, you will have either a heart attack or a stroke, so you can see how important it is to take great care of your blood vessels by having a diet (and herbs) rich in bioflavonoids.

Hawthorn has traditionally been used to reduce blood pressure, but for those with a weak heart, it also supports a natural blood pressure by supporting the heart muscle itself. It strengthens and protects the blood vessel walls from coronary artery disease, and provides the cardiac muscle with extra nutrients, so that it can keep going a few years longer.

🍃 🍃 🍃

Below is a recipe which you can make at home and take a teaspoon of every day to support your heart. If you are on medication, it would be sensible to tell your doctor that you are taking hawthorn honey, but it is unlikely that they will find reason to recommend that you stop.

## HAWTHORN HONEY

🍃 Collect the haws in early autumn, when they are red, ripe and plum.

🍃 Pull them off the twigs and place in a saucepan. Just cover with water and simmer.

🍃 At this point, they develop an unappealing fishy smell. Just ignore that and keep going.

🍃 I add 1 teaspoon of cinnamon per cup of berries to sweeten the taste.

🍃 When the berries are soft, rub them through a sieve so that you have a fine puree.

🍃 The berries are quite starchy, so you may need to add a little water until you get all the pulp through and are left with only pips in your sieve.

🍃 Now add half honey to half puree, and cook down until it reaches a thick toffee-like consistency, then bottle and keep in the fridge.

## Sloes (*Prunus spinosa*)

Although sloes are a well-known and popular berry for flavouring gin, in Britain we are not very familiar with using them as a natural medicine; however, these berries are packed with flavonoids which reduce inflammation in the heart and blood vessels. They have also been found to contain vitamins $B_1$, $B_2$, $B_6$, niacin and folate, which help to reduce homocysteine.[39] High levels of homocysteine are increasingly being recognized as a risk factor for vascular disease. This condition is found when people are deficient in certain B vitamins and folate, and in those who live under stress.

In Eastern Europe, sloes have traditionally been used as a tonic for those who are exhausted and still edgy. They have a relaxing effect on the nerves and a tonic effect on the heart, and so have been used to reinvigorate the body when stamina and resilience are faltering. I would suggest that sloe would make an excellent tonic for post-viral fatigue, particularly when the heart has been injured.

### POST–HEART ATTACK BERRY ELIXIR

Collect hawthorn berries in September and sloes in October/November.

Place in a wide-neck glass jar and cover with red wine. Steep for a month, to extract the flavonoids and healing constituents from the dark fruits, then strain, bottle and drink a small wine glass daily.

If you don't drink alcohol, then steep in red wine vinegar, and when you are ready to drink it, add 4 teaspoons and a little honey to a glass of warm water and enjoy.

## Linden blossom (*Tilia cordata*)

You can lose your head for a moment, as you stand still under a towering linden tree in high summer, for it is an almost narcotic experience. One's senses are overtaken by a powerful perfume and the low resonant hum as you tune into the thousands of bees contentedly collecting the nectar from the insignificant but sweetly scented blossoms.

It is these blossoms which you can collect and dry, to use in a tea to reduce high blood pressure or anxiety. Generations of herb-wise mothers have used this plant for "hysteria". Linden relaxes the nervous system and indeed the involuntary nerves which are embedded within the blood vessel walls.[40] By relaxing and dilating the blood vessels, the blood pressure is mildly reduced, whilst the levels of underlying mind-chatter, which affects us so insidiously, is quietened.

Traditionally, herbalists use *Tilia* for hardening of the arteries, although I cannot find any studies to support this; however, science doesn't always count for everything. Long-term wisdom is sometimes the far better judge of a herb.

## Yarrow (*Achillea millefolium*)

By dilating the blood vessels, yarrow acts in a similar way to linden, but it doesn't carry quite so delightful a fragrance. Yarrow is the warrior's herb, and is a great wound healer. He is a little toughie who can live in the driest of meadows, and still generously gives his flowers to us throughout the summer.

Yarrow is often used by medical herbalists to reduce blood pressure. Raised blood pressure is caused by the heart pumping a bit too hard and/or the blood vessels being a bit too tight. Together this causes an increase of volume and pressure in the blood vessels – hence, increased blood pressure.

So, the aim is to restore the contraction of the heart back to normal, and to open up the blood vessels. In other words, we want to soften the whole cardiovascular system by relaxing it back to its natural state of calm function. Yarrow does both. It calms an overactive heart and dilates the blood vessels, allowing the blood pressure to fall to a healthier state.[41]

**CAUTION:** Yarrow can stimulate the uterus and should not be used by pregnant women.

## Dandelion leaf (*Taraxacum officinale*)

The French, graphically, refer to dandelion as "*pissenlit*", meaning "piss in the bed", which clearly illustrates the action of dandelion leaf. It's a vitamin-rich diuretic, which makes it very helpful in reducing the volume of blood in the blood vessels.

I don't think that it is ideal to take a diuretic constantly, but dandelion leaf and roots are a safe and excellent tonic for the kidneys and liver, and thus act as a cleanser and a refresher to those organ tissues, so that they may function more effectively. By cleansing the liver, there is less congestion in that large gland. All of our blood passes through the liver, which is like a large sponge. When it is congested, it is harder for the blood to pass through, and the backlog of blood can cause pressure on the heart. Cleansing the liver relieves this. By supporting the kidneys, the excess fluid is eliminated more effectively. As a result, the blood pressure is reduced and pressure is again taken off the heart. Taking dandelion leaf for a few weeks in early summer provides the body with a gentle cleansing tonic after a winter of heavier foods.

The leaves are slightly bitter – think of rocket (arugula) and watercress leaves – and tasty in the spring and early summer. Later they become hard and unpleasant to eat, so do pick them at this time of the year and toss into your salad to give your whole system a little cleanse.

## Motherwort (*Leonurus cardiaca*)

The Lion Heart! The botanical name tells you that it is used for the heart, and indeed, *Leonurus* has become one of my favourite herbs to use for those struggling with palpitations of almost any cause. If the Latin doesn't convince you, then perhaps you will heed an old saying: "Drink motherwort tea, and live to a source of continuous astonishment and frustration to waiting heirs."

It is a herbaceous bush which produces tall spikes of tiny pink flowers which the insects love to feed on. In a motherly fashion, she is a prolific producer of viable seeds, which you can share with your friends. Although the flowers are quite insignificant, they are pretty and, when cut down after flowering, will give a second show.

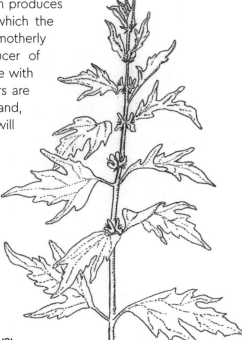

This herb can be used for palpitations related to an overactive thyroid, menopause, anxiety and angina. In the case of anxiety or a mildly overactive thyroid, it works particularly well with *Melissa* (lemon balm).

**CAUTION:** Do avoid motherwort and lemon balm if you have an underactive thyroid.

*♦ ♦ ♦*

*Leonurus* can stimulate the uterus, so should not be used by pregnant women, although the common name of the herb does suggest something slightly different. Motherwort (Mother's herb) has traditionally been used for women in labour, where the contractions are uncoordinated and ineffective. It calms the mother's heart, and almost certainly the baby's too, whilst supporting an effective birthing process. This is something that should be guided by a medical herbalist, midwife or doula familiar with using herbs during labour.

## Olive leaf (*Olea europaea*)
The olive tree is a bit of a miracle tree. The leaves, fruits and oil of the tree contain a compound known as oleuropein, amongst others, which has profoundly beneficial effects on the cardiovascular system. Much of the underlying cause of cardiovascular disease is the result of oxidative inflammatory damage. Olive is potently antioxidant and anti-inflammatory, with particular reference to the arteries.[42]

The inflammatory process damages the blood vessel wall, which is then plugged by fatty cholesterol plaques, but these plugs narrow the arteries, and also represent the weak spot in the blood vessel. With high blood pressure, the weak plaques may rupture, resulting in a blood clot and the high potential for a stroke or heart attack. Olive leaf and oil helps to reduce the inflammation and damage of the blood vessel walls, as well as reduce the fatty plaques and the blood pressure.[43] Combined with hawthorn, you have a very beneficial herbal duo.

## TEA FOR PALPITATIONS OF AN ANXIOUS ORIGIN

🍃 Mix together equal quantities of dried linden blossom, motherwort, vervain and hawthorn leaves and flowers. Store in a tea caddy.

🍃 As required, add 1 teaspoon of this blend to a cup of boiling water and allow to steep for 10 minutes, before straining and drinking.

🍃 **Dosage:** This tea is very safe, and may be taken 3 times a day.

🍃 **CAUTION:** Do not use if pregnant, or if you have an underactive thyroid.

## TEA TO REDUCE BLOOD PRESSURE

If you have been diagnosed with coronary artery disease, it is of the greatest importance that you reconsider your diet. Do see a dietician or nutritionist to this end. Then with a healthy diet and exercise, this homemade tea may possibly save your life. It is quite safe to use with your doctor's medication, but it would be prudent and only polite to let your doctor know which herbs you are using.

hawthorn leaves, flowers and berries
yarrow and/or linden blossom
dandelion leaf
olive leaf

🍃 Mix together equal parts of the dried components of the plants listed, and store in an airtight container.

🍃 Add 1 teaspoon of the tea to a cup of boiling water and allow to steep for 10 minutes before straining. Drink twice a day.

## A SALAD OF LOVE FOR YOUR HEART

rocket (arugula) and watercress leaves (decongest the liver)

dandelion leaves (diuretic)

hawthorn flowers and young leaves (cardiac support)

black grapes (rich in flavonoids)

blueberries (rich in flavonoids)

smoked mackerel (omega-3)

beetroot (beets) (reduces blood pressure)

dressing of olive oil, lemon juice and garlic (decongests the liver and reduces blood pressure and cholesterol levels)

# Horse chestnut (*Aesculus hippocastanum*)

Besides conker competitions, there is another great way to use the seeds of this stunningly beautiful tree. Within the fat conkers is a constituent called aescin, which strengthens and protects, particularly the veins. This is important: where hawthorn and olive are indicated for the arteries, horse chestnut is indicated for the veins.

# VARICOSE VEINS

Varicose veins occur when the vessels have become so engorged and distended that the valves no longer work effectively to keep the blood moving upward toward the heart. Instead the blood tends to puddle down at the ankles, putting further pressure on the veins and causing even more distension. It is almost a losing battle – that is, until you seek the help of horse chestnut.

The horse-chestnut seed has a very special action on the veins. It strengthens the integrity of the blood vessel wall, tightening the distended veins and healing the cellular structure so that it is no longer leaky. In this way the herb significantly reduces the puffiness and swelling around the ankles. By alleviating the congested and stagnant blood which pools at the ankles, the danger of varicose ulcers is much abated. Even if someone has varicose ulcers, horse chestnut would be a herb to consider, but this must be prescribed by a medical herbalist because it would need an internal prescription with other herbs to support the action.

Whilst horse chestnut is a wonderful herb it does have some slightly toxic effects on the gut, and so for the lay person, it is much safer to use this herb only externally, and not internally as may be employed by a medical herbalist. Thankfully, you can make an excellent horse-chestnut gel to apply directly to your legs.

## HORSE-CHESTNUT GEL

**To make this gel, you must first make a tincture of horse chestnuts.**

🌿 Collect 2 handfuls of fresh conkers, and smash them up with a hammer. Now put these into a glass Kilner clip-top jar and pour pure vodka over the seeds, so that the alcohol just covers the smashed conkers. Leave them to extract for 2 weeks. Once the 2 weeks have passed, strain the tincture through muslin and store in a glass bottle in a dark cupboard.

**To make your gel:**

🌿 Purchase 500g (1lb 2oz) of aloe vera gel, and scoop it out into a ceramic bowl.

🌿 Slowly add 50ml (1¾fl oz) of your tincture, all the time whisking the fluid into the gel.

🌿 Now add 5ml of cypress essential oil, and whisk thoroughly into the gel.

🌿 Seal this gel in a screw-top container, and you can apply it to your legs every day to tighten and soothe varicose veins.

🌿 Do not use this gel on broken skin. If you have a varicose ulcer, you can use this gel around the area, but not over the ulcer itself.

**There are other things that you can do to ease the discomfort of varicose veins:**

- Place a thick book or a thinnish cushion under the foot of your mattress, so that while you are sleeping, your legs are slightly elevated, helping to drain the blood back up to your heart.

- Twice a day, rinse your lower legs alternately with warm then cold water – always ending with cold water, so that the muscles of your veins relax and contract. This is like a little exercise regime for your veins.

- Raise your legs above the level of your heart several times a day to drain the blood from your legs. This could be done after you have applied your homemade horse-chestnut gel, to allow it to sink into the tissues. Lie back on the sofa with your ankles propped on the sofa arms, or if you are more supple, lie on the floor with your bottom pressed against a wall and your legs raised up against the wall. This is quite comfortable, and I am told by my yoga teacher that it is good for the brain!

- Eat at least one handful of blueberries or blackberries every day, have a glass of red wine, and nibble a square or two of very dark chocolate to provide your veins with the flavonoids necessary to strengthen their walls. Make sure that you eat plenty of dark-skinned vegetables and fruits.

- Do go for walks because the blood is pumped uphill by the contraction of your calf muscles squidging the blood upward. If you walk, you help to relieve the puddling of the blood in your ankles. When you get home, you can raise your legs for 10–20 minutes to further help to drain the legs of too much blood.

# Oak leaves (*Quercus robur*)

For those suffering from haemorrhoids (piles), conkers are very helpful, but so too are oak leaves. The reason we use oak is for the tannins, which are astringent in their actions. This means that they tighten engorged tissues, like piles, and stop bleeding. The conkers are rich in saponins which are anti-inflammatory and tighten blood vessel walls, so together conkers and oak are a winning combination. The original idea was to use oak bark, but that involves harming the tree, and although you could collect some twigs and scrape the bark off, that does seem like a lot of work. Oak leaves are particularly rich in tannins in September, so this is a great time to collect a bag of oak leaves and dry them for use throughout the year.

Conkers have the habit of quickly becoming fungal, so I like to smash them up and dry them slowly in an oven, then store them in a brown paper bag. The oak leaves can be dried over a day or so in a warm shed or cupboard.

Tannins and saponins are both water soluble, which means that they can be extracted in a teapot and poured into your bath, or you can make a little pad to press against the piles.

> Oak leaves are particularly rich in tannins in September, so this is a great time to collect a bag of oak leaves and dry them for use throughout the year.

## CONKER AND OAK-LEAF BATH

This bath would be beneficial for both varicose veins and haemorrhoids, and will certainly bring relief, but since it is more diluted than the gel, the effect will be milder.

Add 2 dessertspoons of crushed conkers and 1 handful of oak leaves to a teapot.

Fill with boiling water and leave to extract for 4 hours, or even overnight.

When you are ready for a bath, strain and pour this into your bath.

If you don't have a bath, or your haemorrhoids are in a flare-up phase, you can pour this infusion over some small sanitary pads and place these in a plastic container in the refrigerator. When you feel the need, take one out and press against the piles for immediate relief.

Haemorrhoids are caused by straining, so it is of the utmost importance that your diet contains enough roughage and olive oil to maintain a soft stool. In that way, you keep your piles quiet.

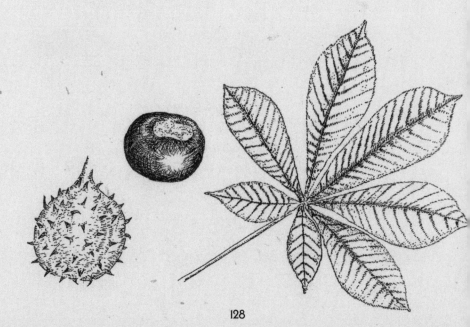

## A WITCH'S LOVE POTION

When we consider affairs of the heart, we cannot ignore the emotional heart, and our desire to be loved. Throughout the ages, love potions have been the mainstay of many a witch's financial stability, and I thought you may be interested in two old love spells.

## LOVE SPELL NO. 1

Mix together vervain (dedicated to Venus, Goddess of Love), the seeds and flowers of elecampane (the herb of the elves) and mistletoe berries (sperm of the gods), and dry in the oven until they are crisp.

Pound these into a powder, and add a teaspoon to the wine of your beloved, who shall instantly fall in love with you!

## LOVE SPELL NO. 2

Another, potentially less successful, love potion entails tying a little bag around your neck containing vervain and a dried-out toad.

*When we consider affairs of the heart, we cannot ignore the emotional heart, and our desire to be loved.*

# CHAPTER 5

## The Summer Solstice and the Oak King

In Celtic mythology, the eternal battle between light and dark is expressed though the mythological Oak King who represents summer, and the Holly King who presides over winter. The high point of the solar journey through the year is the Summer Solstice, when the days are longest and the nights are shortest.

On the Summer Solstice, the very day that the Oak King reaches the zenith of his power, he is slain by the Holly King. Imperceptibly at first, as the days grow shorter his strength fades, as day by day the power of the Holly King grows. So, too, at the Winter Solstice, when the Holly King, at the height of his power, roars his victory, he in turn is slain by the Oak King. On and on through the aeons of time this battle wages, never ending.

For now, we are focussing on the Summer Solstice, represented by the mighty oak. The Druids call him Duir. He is the king of the forest, and in all cultures the oak represents strength, protection, steadfastness. He is a single organism and a living city, home to over 300 species of plant, insect, bird and mammal. This is a tree that we can lean against when we feel weak, in need of solace, a quiet place to think or just to be. The mighty oak is the tree we turn to for strength and courage.

It is venerated by the major cultures of Europe, and sacred to Zeus, Jupiter, Dagda and Thor – each of these gods had dominion over rain, thunder and lightning. As one of the tallest trees in the forest, with a high starch content, the venerable oak is an excellent conductor of electricity and thus often victim to lightning strikes. I remember once walking in the forest and being absolutely astonished as I came across a huge oak, exploded to pieces. The shockwaves still resonated in the atmosphere.

Like a good king, the oak sacrifices himself by standing in front of danger and protecting his family of smaller trees by taking the hit. A massive discharge of negative ions, channelled into the earth, brings fertility to the surrounding land, and crops grow abundantly for years afterwards. It might cut him down, but sometimes the following year, fresh supple shoots regrow, thus he reinvents himself. This is the wisdom of the mighty oak and the blasted oak.

# HOT AND ITCHY CONDITIONS

🌿 ELDERFLOWERS 🌿 RIBWORT
🌿 NETTLE LEAVES 🌿 THYME 🌿 CORNSILK

For most of us, summer is a joyful time, where we can enjoy being outside in nature. Many, however, find it a time of misery as they suffer with the red itchy eyes and streaming noses of hay fever. For others, the heat brings on yeast infections or urinary tract infections. All these hot and itchy conditions can make summer more difficult than winter, but often our lovely herbs can make a big difference.

## HAY FEVER

### Elderflowers (*Sambucus nigra*)

I remember one day attending a workshop in the Sussex countryside, when hay fever suddenly struck. My nose poured like a tap, making it impossible to concentrate on the fascinating demonstration. In desperation, I cast my eyes outside and spied an elder tree in full bloom. I managed to get a cup of boiling water from the kitchen and dropped an inflorescence (a whole flower head) of elder into the mug. Inhaling the fragrant steam immediately soothed my prickling nasal passages, and as soon as I drank the infusion, my hay fever halted. It was like magic! Two hours later, the tap turned on again, and I repeated the infusion, and again the benevolence of the elder saved my day.

Benevolence indeed, for every year, just as the hay fever season strikes, millions of elder trees burst into bloom like a creamy cappuccino froth across the land, and it is toward these lacy flowers that we may turn for relief. Elderflowers have an anti-inflammatory effect on the mucous membranes. In the late summer, the ovaries of flowers ripen into blue-black berries, bursting with vitamin C and antiviral properties, just as we need the immune boost to ward off early winter viruses.

## Ribwort (*Plantago lanceolata and P. ovata*)

Ribwort can be found every-where, as the charm opposite tells us. It is found in every meadow, along every country path, and down any city alley. It is so common that it is despised, but despise it not, for this is a plant of power and respite.

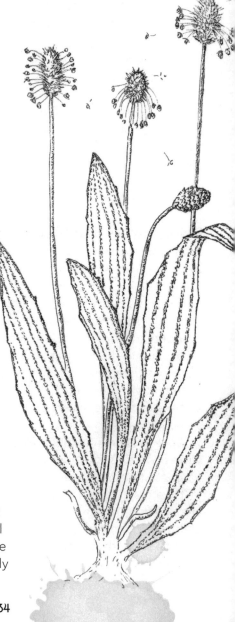

*Plantago* is classed by herbalists as a refrigerant. This means that it cools hot and inflamed tissues. As a gentle astringent, it tightens engorged and inflamed tissues, but it is also a demulcent, soothing raw and sore tissues. Ribwort has a particular affinity for the mucous membranes and I love to use it for the nasal passages, the bronchi, the bladder wall and sometimes the stomach.[44]

Ribwort is a simple hay-fever remedy. Do be a bit careful, because some people are allergic to the pollen, but I have never known anyone have a reaction to the leaf. The simplest way to use ribwort, or waybread if you prefer its ancient name, is simply to pluck a leaf and chew it. Make sure that you chew the leaf, sucking out all the juices, and then spit out the hard ribs. You will find that it quickly

*And you, Waybread, mother of herbs,*
*eastward open, mighty inside.*
*Over you chariots creaked, over you queens rode,*
*over you brides cried out, over you bulls snorted.*
*All of these, you withstood, and dashed against.*
*As you withstand poison and that which flies*
*and the loathsome foe that roves the land.*

From the "Nine Herbs Charm",
as recorded in the 10th-century *Lacnunga*

soothes streaming hay fever. It is not the most delicious taste, but when the juices are in the mouth, they quickly dissolve through the thin tissues of your mouth cavity into the bloodstream, which is why you really need to chew and suck those juices.

This herb is useful also for those hard, dry coughs which leave your airways so raw and irritated that this in itself perpetuates the cough, and a vicious cycle ensues. In this case, you might prefer to make a tea and add some honey to soothe the mucous membranes.

Ribwort is an excellent remedy for insect and nettle stings, and far more effective than dock leaf. If you are stung by a nettle, you will inevitably find ribwort growing in close proximity. Pluck a leaf, chew it into a paste and rub onto the sting, and the pain will go immediately. It is quite an extraordinary experience because you can feel the buzz of the nettle sting, but no pain.

If you have come out in hives, drink plantago tea. Collect five or six leaves, rinse off and drop into a cup of boiling water, then drink. You can even gently wipe the affected area with the infusion. This simple remedy would be further enhanced by adding a few mint leaves, for their cooling effect.

## Nettle leaves (*Urtica dioica*)

The word "nettle" comes from the Anglo-Saxon word "*noedl*", which means "needle", and indeed you don't even need a microscope to see the brittle, glass-like needles growing out of the leaf in fierce self-defence. The needles carry histamine, and thus it is an irony that this very leaf is used for the treatment of a histamine reaction, such as hay fever or hives.

These fierce friends are rather fabulous at alleviating an allergic reaction. Scientists have discovered that they have at least a three-pronged attack, by inhibiting or blocking histamine release, inhibiting the breakdown of mast cells in the blood, and inhibiting prostaglandin release – all inflammatory molecules which stimulate an allergic reaction.[45]

## Thyme (*Thymus vulgaris*)

Thyme is a natural antibacterial and antifungal herb, and may be used either fresh or dried.[46] It is particularly helpful for congested sinuses which can become excruciatingly tender. Sometimes the tissues lining the sinus cavity can swell so much that the mucus becomes stuck, and infection can breed, so it is important to disinfect the sinus cavities, reduce the inflammation and drain the thick sticky mucus.

To this end you can consider thyme and ribwort to disinfect the sinuses, elderflowers and ribwort to reduce the inflammation, and either horseradish or chilli to flush the sinus cavity (think hot curry!).

These fierce friends are rather fabulous at alleviating an allergic reaction. Scientists have discovered that they have at least a three-pronged attack ...

## HAY FEVER TEA

**By combining elderflowers, ribwort and nettle leaf, you have an excellent first aid kit for the home treatment of hay fever. It is so good that you may not need anything else.**

🌿 Dry equal portions of nettle leaf, ribwort leaf and elderflowers. Mix together and store in a tea tin.

🌿 When required, add 1 teaspoon of the blend to a cup of boiling water. Try to inhale the steam through your nose to gain the most benefits possible, then drink when cool enough.

🌿 If you are using fresh plants, then 2 teaspoons per cup is the dose.

🌿 All these herbs are quite safe, and this tea can be taken every 2–3 hours, as required during the day.

🌿 You might even like to make larger quantities and freeze into ice cubes, which can be sucked or dropped into cool water, to use as required.

## TEA FOR A SINUS INFECTION

1 tsp fresh thyme or ½ tsp dried
    (kitchen cupboard) thyme
1 tsp chopped ribwort
1 elderflower inflorescence
    (complete flower head)
a large pinch of hot chilli powder

🌿 Put all of this into a teapot, and drink as hot as you are able to, without scalding your mouth. Drink 1 cup every 2 hours.

# SORE, ITCHY EYES

The membranes of the eyes can really be affected by pollen, and the temptation to rub is almost irresistible. Of course, the more you rub, the more they swell. This can quickly be relieved with a cold, mildly astringent infusion. Black tea leaves (your leftover tea bags) make an excellent first aid option, because black tea is rich in tannins which calm the inflamed tissues, and the bags are perfect to plop over the eyes. If you want to be a little more exotic, you can collect some leaves and flowers from your garden or allotment.

We visited friends one summer's day, and their lovely little dog had swollen red eyes. They called it "sausage eyes" because every summer his little eyelids would swell so much that they looked like tiny sausages. My friends had an enviable vegetable garden with huge fruit cages, and within those cages were strawberry plants. The leaves of strawberries and blackberries are rich in tannins, and both have been traditionally used to treat sore eyes. Sue made an infusion of strawberry leaves and gently wiped her dog's eyes, and she sent me a delighted message to say that it had worked a treat!

## INFUSION FOR HAY-FEVER EYES

1 tsp chopped ribwort leaves
2 tsp chopped bramble or
    strawberry leaves
½ tsp chopped mint leaves

Rinse the herbs, then add ½ cup boiling water and steep for 30 minutes. Strain through a double layer of muslin, then dip a cotton wool pad in the infusion and lightly squeeze. Now take a few minutes to lie down while you gently press the soaked pads over your eyes.

# INSECT BITES AND STINGS

My absolute number one remedy emergency for bites and stings is ribwort. As soon as you have been stung by an insect, pluck a ribwort leaf, chew it into a paste, and press it onto the sting like a little compress. This will give immediate relief.

*   *   *

Below is another, slightly more elegant option for bites and stings:

~~~~~~~~~~~~~~~~~~~~~~~~~~~~~~~~~~~~~~~~~~~~~

**ALOE AND TURMERIC GEL**

**You can make a pot of this gel and keep it in the refrigerator for bites and stings.**

50g (1¾oz) aloe vera gel

1 heaped tsp turmeric powder

3 drops of peppermint essential oil

5 drops of sweet birch essential oil
(do not use if you are allergic to salicylates or aspirin)

20 drops of lavender essential oil

Mix all the ingredients together and dab on the burn or sting. Do not use this on open wounds – only apply if the skin hasn't broken.

~~~~~~~~~~~~~~~~~~~~~~~~~~~~~~~~~~~~~~~~~~~~~

# LOCALIZED YEAST AND FUNGAL CONDITIONS

Sometimes antibiotics are very helpful and can save lives, but it is well known that they are over-prescribed and frequently quite unnecessary. Far better to build a robust immune system with herbs and nutritional supplements, and use natural medicines to fight infection if required. The health cost of using antibiotics on our body system can be severe.

Yeast and fungal conditions come from inside our body. It is not so much an infection as an environmental imbalance, where usually too much sugar and an imbalanced gut biome or hormonal imbalance encourages yeast to overgrow. You can find further information on this in Chapter 5. Having said that, sometimes yeasts don't bother us unless it is very hot, and thus remain localized problems. For conditions such as these, please see below.

## Fungal toenails

Most people wear shoes and socks all day and every day, but because feet perspire, shoes provide a warm, moist and dark environment for the fungus to thrive. If you wish to clear athlete's foot, it is important to thoroughly dry your feet after a shower, and then hot-wash that towel after every use. To save water, perhaps keep a small hand towel for feet, and use larger towels for the rest of your body.

The fungal spores live in your socks and shoes. It is sometimes worth throwing out all your socks and starting with new cotton or woollen socks. While it is not practical to do this with shoes, you can try not to wear the same shoes every day, and shake an antifungal powder into your shoes before and after you put them on, remembering that yeasts love a moist environment, so you need to keep the environment powder-dry.

If your nails are very fungal, you can apply neat tea tree or palmarosa essential oil underneath the nail once a day. You will need to do this for months, and it is worthwhile alternating the oils weekly so that the yeast doesn't develop resistance.

## Yeast rashes under the breasts and in the groin area

When skin rests against skin, it is natural that warmth and perspiration create a damp environment. This is why men often suffer from "jock itch" in the groin area, and women with large breasts can develop rashes under their bust line. Both sexes can have skin yeast infections under their arms or any area of the body where skin on skin is generating heat and moisture. The antifungal powder recipe below is deliciously fresh smelling, but also cooling and drying. It significantly diminishes yeast skin infections. Apply twice a day at least.

## ANTIFUNGAL POWDER

250g (9oz) cornflour (cornstarch)
250g (9oz) bentonite clay
20 drops of palmarosa essential oil
20 drops of lemongrass essential oil
20 drops of tea tree essential oil
20 drops of geranium essential oil

Combine in a bowl and mix with a balloon whisk. The oils will knock back bacteria and yeasts, and the clay is cooling and absorbent of perspiration and moisture. It also makes a fantastic deodorant under the arms.

# Yeast bladder infections

Over my years as a medical herbalist, I have seen and treated many women with this problem, which presents as cystitis, with pain and discomfort in the bladder, but does not respond to antibiotics. Bladders prefer teas (or infusions) over tinctures, and the herbal tea below is very helpful because the herbs are both antibacterial and antifungal.

This infusion is appropriate for normal cystitis, as well as a yeast bladder infection, as a first step in the treatment process. If you do not feel better within two days, please consult a professional.

## SAGE, CALENDULA AND THYME TEA

1 tsp fresh thyme, or ½ tsp
    dried thyme
1 tsp fresh chopped garden sage,
    or ½ tsp dried sage
3 calendula flowers (fresh or dried)
4 leaves of ribwort

Put the herbs into a teapot and add a cup of boiling water. Quickly put on the lid and allow to draw for 5 minutes, then drink while warm. Do this 3 times a day.

**CAUTION:** Do not use sage if you are prone to epilepsy.

## Thrush

Thrush occurs mainly in the mouth, vagina, under the foreskin, and anal areas. To treat oral thrush, use the tea above. The vaginal, penis and anal thrush can be treated slightly differently.

An itchy bottom, or anal thrush, is not the sort of topic one generally brings up in conversation, but it is extremely common. For most cases, there is a very simple remedy – give up sugar and the itchiness will go. It is that simple.

The problem with vaginal thrush is that the delicate environment of local bacteria has been disturbed or destroyed, giving the yeast an opportunity to proliferate. Antibiotics not only kill the bacteria which cause various infections, but also the trillions of friendly bacteria which live in our body and serve useful purposes.

Women who suffer from thrush can help to re-establish the bacterial population by using live plain yogurt. The healthy vaginal bacterial population is dominated mainly by *Lactobacillus* species, and the same bacteria are found in this yogurt. It is an old-fashioned remedy to inoculate the vagina with yogurt, and you can see the wisdom of that practice. This is most simply achieved by dipping a small tampon into a little yogurt, then inserting into the vagina. Remove the tampon after 10 minutes, and repeat this at night.

Women naturally have an acidic environment in their vagina, whilst the male sperm is alkaline. Thus, post sex, when the man has ejaculated into the vagina, the pH changes to be more alkaline and conducive to yeast flourishing. I advise my patients who suffer from this problem as follows: both partners must be treated because the yeast is passed back and forth between the couple. So, following sex, she should douche her vagina with a diluted solution of apple cider vinegar (1 tsp apple cider vinegar, 1 drop of geranium essential oil or tea tree oil, 1 cup of tepid warm water) to wash out the sperm and re-establish the acid environment. Of course, if you are trying to become pregnant then this should not be done. The man can wash his penis with the same liquid.

## Cornsilk (*Zea mays*)

Cornsilk is a natural diuretic and anti-inflammatory with a particular affinity for the mucous membranes of the urinary tract. By inhibiting the attachment of bacteria to the bladder wall, cornsilk helps to prevent and alleviate bladder infections.[47]

When the kidneys are stimulated to flush, the bacteria are washed out of the bladder, but also, do bear in mind that the diuretic action can lower the blood pressure, so keep your water intake up. It is also interesting that the polysaccharides (natural sugars) of the herb have been shown to significantly reduce blood sugar and cholesterol levels. Be aware that if you are already using blood-sugar or blood-pressure medication that cornsilk may exacerbate the effect, so use with restraint and some caution.

All you need to do is peel the cornsilk off your sweetcorn and allow it to dry until you need to use it. Once dried, it can be stored in a glass jar, where it looks like a little nest. Simply drop a nest into a cup of boiling water when you need to.

### EMERGENCY TEA FOR CYSTITIS

1 tsp chopped ribwort
1 tsp fresh thyme or ½ tsp
    dried thyme
3–4 fresh marshmallow leaves
1 nest of cornsilk
1 calendula flower

Put the herbs in a cup of boiling water. Steep until cool enough to drink. Take this tea 4 times a day, and see a herbalist or doctor if your symptoms haven't resolved within 2 days.

# CHAPTER 6

## Lughnasadh and Harvesting with Love

# A TiME OF HARVEST

### 🍃 HOPS 🍃 LAVENDER 🍃 SLIPPERY ELM
### 🍃 CABBAGE 🍃 GARLIC 🍃 CAROB

Lughnasadh – the time of gathering in. It is the season when our endeavours over the spring and summer have blossomed, swollen, ripened and now fruited. In the countryside, this is the time when the fruits and grains from the fields are gathered in and brought to the safety of the barns, where they are stored for the coming winter. In our case, this is when we gather the fruits and roots from the hedgerows and our gardens to turn into medicines for the coming winter and the following year.

Just as we have life cycles, circadian cycles and menstrual cycles, so too does the Earth have her cycles, and it is wise to work with these cycles if we wish to most benefit from her gifts.

During the winter, the vital force of the plant is contracted and safely curled up, deep within the Earth, where it rests and gathers strength. Then, as the sun starts to strengthen, it draws the life-force of the earth through the plants upward, and so they grow. The spring and early summer is the time when the life-force is surging up through the tips of the leaves and shoots. This is when we harvest the soft green detoxing leaves such as nettles, clivers, ground elder, willow and birch, because the strength of the plant is in the shoots and leaf tips.

As the season slips into early summer, the strength of the plants continues to expand, branching out, with flowers budding and opening. This is the time to harvest flowering plants such as roses, calendula, feverfew, St John's wort, motherwort and marshmallow leaves.

The summer gets hotter and reaches its zenith in July and August. At this time, the volatile oils are at their most potent. These are found in the herbs which carry fragrance within their leaves and flowers, such as hyssop, thyme, rosemary, sage, lavender, rose geranium, lemon balm and hops cones. At this time, we also harvest the leaves which needed to be strengthened by the sun such as oak leaves, yarrow and rue.

In the late summer, the ovaries of the flowers which were fertilized around Beltane have now swollen with the warmth of the summer days, and are ready to pick. Rosehips, haws, blackberries, horse chestnuts and chestnuts, and much later, sloes.

After the height of summer, the Oak King starts to die, and the cycle of energy naturally descends slowly back down into the earth. The plants have spent all summer absorbing the goodness of the sun's rays, and now these photosynthesized nutrients are transported downward and stored in the roots. At this time, the roots swell with starches and healing constituents, and so this is the time when the roots are at their most potent. Thus, we harvest herbs like elecampane, burdock and marshmallow root.

Harvesting by the cycles of the year can be further refined when you harvest according to the cycles of the moon. The Moon and the Earth act like magnets to each other. The Moon tries to pull the Earth toward her. One could romantically propose that might be because the Moon was once part of the Earth and they used to share a magnetic field. The gravitational force of the moon has a powerful effect on all the waters of the Earth. When the moon waxes, it draws the water toward itself, and when she is waning, the forces have a relaxing effect on the Earth. Thus, because the waters of the plant are drawn upward during a new or full moon, this is the time to harvest above-ground plant material. As the moon wanes, the gravitational force is lessened, and so the waters of the plant descend, thus below-ground plant material is harvested at the waning of the moon.

If you are inclined, you can even further refine this by harvesting according to the daily sun cycle. Again, the energies rise in the morning, and sink from noon till sunset. As such, you can capture the best strength of the plant by harvesting all plant parts above the ground after the dew has dried until noon. Then from noon until sunrise, you can harvest all parts below the ground level.

So, as an example, a gypsy friend told me that they harvest lawn daisies in the early morning, in June, under the sign of Cancer, when the moon is full. Apart from the magical aspects, we can see why these wise folk, who live close to the land, might harvest as such.

## Practicalities when harvesting:

- Be respectful to the plant being whose limbs you are removing for your own benefit. Weird though it may feel, do ask permission – you will be surprised to find that sometimes you are refused, or guided elsewhere.

- Always leave much more than you take; i.e. don't take everything.

- Collect away from polluted roads, in as clean an area as possible.

- Be conscious of areas where dogs or foxes may lift their legs.

- Harvest leaves and flowers once the dew has dried, so that there is less chance of mould developing.

- Spread your harvest out for a few hours to allow the insects to escape.

- Always thank the plants whilst you are harvesting. Think of it as a benevolent being of power rather than a green static thing in your garden.

- Herbs can be dried by tying them into small bundles and hanging from the ceiling. Or by spreading out on wired trays or even a tray covered in newspaper or a clean cotton dish towel.

- Make sure all the plant matter is absolutely dry before storing in paper bags, unless you are going to process it into a tincture or syrup. If it is not completely dry, it will turn mouldy. If it does become mouldy, you must throw it away because mould can become toxic.

- Roots are best preserved if they are sliced into thin strips, so that they dry completely.

- Aromatic herbs should be dried in the shade or a cool, dry area. If the area is too hot, you will lose the volatile oils to the atmosphere and end up with a weak herb to work with.

- Store your dried herbs or herbal medicines in a cool, dark place. They will usually keep for about a year.

# A PERSONAL EXPERIENCE OF LISTENING To PLANTS

I love the way plants teach me. One morning, I was in my garden, harvesting verbascum (mullein) in the usual way by plucking the flowers off the stem, when suddenly I had a strong feeling that the plant finds this a rather brutal method (quite right!). It was suggested that if I were to gently shake the stem, verbascum would be generous. Well, of course, I did just that, and to my disappointment, not many flowers fell. But then, after only a second or two, many flowers gently dropped off the stem onto the earth. Gifted, not taken. I like that.

## HARVESTING HERBS AS SENTIENT BEINGS

My apothecary garden is a community of sentient beings. The plants are the main players, but the birds, the furry creatures, the horses over the hedge, the cows in the far field, the human visitors and I, all contribute to the overall sense of harmony and contentment within that small space.

This harmony, I hope, is conferred to my patients through the energy of the medicines, and of course, the quality of the products, hand harvested, at their peak of power, with love. So, what does that mean?

I think it boils down to respect and consideration for all the beings, seen and unseen, of my garden. Every living being lives to express itself freely, thus the first rule of herb harvesting is that you leave more than you take, and in this way, the plant can complete its life cycle by flowering, seeding and feeding the bees and butterflies. Perhaps it delights a flower to be tickled by a bumble bee, and for the bees, it appears to be a narcotic experience as they bumble from flower to flower in an apparent drunken blur of busy bliss. Total focus. They are in flow. Doing their thing. Probably not ruminating on Fenella the bee who stole their flower.

I take this sentience to the level where I ask the plant to show me which flowers, etc. I may take, and whilst this might seem quite ridiculous, I am aware that some flowers glow at me, while others push me away. I learnt this originally from nettles, who would gently sting me, and then I knew that it was time to move along. Over the years, my sensitivity to the plant world develops.

It is easy to drop a twiglet when harvesting, but out of respect, I always pick it up, because it is not right to waste a miracle – for what is a plant who can heal us but a miracle? It is the ultimate magic when you take a weed, extract it, and give it to a sick human, and their health is fully recovered. Alchemy and transformation. Such power should be respected.

If at all possible, I don't harvest a flower upon which an insect is feeding. Can you imagine having your larder raided by some enormous troll?

Once the plant has been harvested, I leave the herb out for a few hours for the hidden insects to escape, for it is amazing how many tinies live amongst the petals. I often think what a wonderful life it must be to sleep snug in the silky petals of a fragrant rose. Your entire world a universe of perfume. Think of the light through the petals as the sun rises. What about the prisms of light showering your world from the dew?

The herb is then either extracted as a tincture, or dried and cut up for herbal infusions. It always makes me sad when I hang marshmallow or Californian poppies to dry, because for a few days their petals open and close with the sun. Toward the end of summer, when I harvest bunches of plants, and lay them out on the lawn before tying them into bundles, again, it makes me sad, for they look like animals which have been hunted; however, I do pay the plants in the best way I can think of.

In the autumn, I put my plants to bed, tucked under a thick layer of manure or compost, so that they can rest and be fed over the dark, cold winter months in the safety of Mother Earth. But this offering is so mundane when compared to that of the ancients.

As an example, although it is tradition to offer a libation of honey when harvesting vervain, the ancient Druids were far more meticulous when it came to honouring their harvested herbs. Great ceremonies were conducted at specific times of the day and the year, and in a precise ritual. According to Pliny, the Druids harvested vervain at the rising of the Dog Star, Sirius (which rises in July and August), this being the height of summer and indeed an excellent time to cut vervain. They would harvest when neither the sun nor the moon were in the sky, so as not to offend the planets by having to witness the sacred herb being cut. Before they harvested, an offering of honeycomb was given to the Earth as a token of amends for the "violence and wrongs of depriving her of so sacred a herb". The herb was then cut without the use of iron, and held aloft in the left hand.

The Druidesses had their own rituals for harvesting vervain. They would not even touch so sacred a herb. At midnight on the full moon, a long rope with a loop was thrown around the plant, and then tied to the big toe of a virgin who had to pull the rope (with her toe) until the plant was uprooted. The eldest Druidesses then received the plant in a cloth, and carried it home in reverence.

Other herbs were harvested in fear and it's said that the mandrake plant will scream if uprooted. If the harvester hears that scream, he shall surely die. To avert such an outcome, a stray dog was caught and a rope was tied around its neck and the stalk of the plant. It would then be lured by a piece of meat, whilst the harvesters would cover their ears. While going for the meat, the dog would uproot the plant, and no doubt later die from the deadly screams of Mandragora.

## HARVESTING A VIKING'S HOARD OF CONKERS

Not many people would consider a basketful of conkers to be a treasure trove, but we should, for gold is cold, and plants can heal. What good is wealth without wellness? Holistic wellness is much more than simply not being sick. It must also include our mental, emotional and spiritual wellbeing, which in turn may derive from a sense of freedom to be oneself, self-empowerment and a sense of peace with who we are, and those in our life. Expressing our unique creativity and shining that creative enlightenment out to the world enriches the whole of society. For many people, working with plants as medicine, as food, as cosmetics or perfumes, as fabric dyes, as something to weave, or teaching children to grow vegetables is their way of expressing their creativity, or just having some good old-fashioned fun. Wellness becomes deep wealth when one's life becomes a tapestry of richness.

Therefore, as something fun to do, you might like to make soap out of conkers. There is much on the internet which tells us that conkers were used by the Vikings to make soap, but alas, that just is not true. Horse-chestnut trees come from the Balkan peninsula, and only migrated to the rest of Europe around the 17th century.

Nonetheless, conkers do make a rather fabulous soap, and that is because they are rich in saponins. The word is derived from the Latin word "*sapo*", which means "soap", or "to lather", and indeed, these plant constituents do produce a lather. Saponins are very common in the plant world, and I am often reminded of their presence when I shake up a demijohn of tincture, which can produce quite a lather. Horse-chestnut seeds (conkers) are rich in saponins, and as such have been used for centuries for washing hair and fabric.

## CONKER LAUNDRY LIQUID

🌿 To make completely natural laundry liquid, you collect about 12 conkers and bash them up in a cast iron mortar and pestle, or you could wrap them in a clean cloth and smash them with a hammer.

🌿 Now place the crushed conkers in a saucepan with some hot water and leave to extract overnight. In the morning, the water will have turned milky white. Strain the conkers from the liquid and add some lavender essential oil if you wish before you use the liquid to wash a load of linen. This is a great option for those who have allergies to washing powders.

🌿 If you want to use the conkers throughout the year, simply collect a Viking's hoard of conkers, crush them and dry at a low heat in the oven, then store in a glass jar. Use half a cup per load of washing. It will save you a small fortune.

# YOUR CAULDRON OF NOURISHMENT

Our digestive system is a tube which runs from mouth to anus, and miraculously, somewhere along that nine-metre pipeline, food is taken in and broken down into nutrient molecules which are absorbed into the bloodstream, toxins are separated out and the waste matter is removed – all in one long tube! Our bodies are unsung miracles.

An old homeopath friend of mine used to say that in order to bring someone back to full health, you must start with their core. In other words, the digestive system must be functioning optimally, for how can someone be well if their intestine is so inflamed that undigested molecules escape into the bloodstream, the major organs of waste elimination are blocked, and they are unable to fully digest and absorb their nutrients?

I like to use the analogy of a flowing stream, which can become a stagnant pond if clogged up with debris and pollution. Slime soon covers the surface of the pond, and the water becomes fetid. The cure is not to add endless chemicals to kill the algae, but to unblock the entry and exit points of the pond so that the stale water can flow out, replaced with fresh water. In this way a healthy stream is re-established, and the environment both in the stream and surrounding area can be restored. The result is a flourishing ecosystem.

Our bodies are more of a collective ecosystem of intelligent cells and friendly bacteria than a single individual organism, and so we need to treat ourselves as we would a garden by feeding our digestive system with healthy organic food, and making sure that the streams of elimination are flowing cleanly, so that the whole community works together in harmony.

For you to benefit from your food properly, you need sufficient hydrochloric acid in your stomach and enzymes in your small intestine to digest your food. This requires a calm nervous system, for if you are in the fight-or-flight sympathetic nervous state, your digestive processes are switched off.

Once the food has been broken down by sufficient mastication and enzymatic cleaving, the nutrients are absorbed by the intestinal wall into the inner environment of the bloodstream. The blood runs through our sponge-like liver, where toxins are removed and packed off to the kidneys and bowel, whilst the nutrients are transported to the cells which require them. The bowels are hopefully working efficiently and remove the toxins from the body.

# NATURAL DIGESTIVE ENZYMES

Our nervous system is divided into the voluntary nervous system, where we decide to move a finger, and the involuntary nervous system, which regulates the life processes that we don't think about, such as breathing, digestion, etc. The involuntary nervous system is further divided into the sympathetic nervous system (fight or flight) and the parasympathetic nervous system (rest and digest).

The parasympathetic nervous system is engaged when we feel calm, relaxed and happy. This is the ideal state for the body to secrete the enzymes necessary for the proper digestion of our food. However, if we are upset, in a hurry or living in a stressful environment, we are in sympathetic dominance and our food cannot be correctly digested. The sympathetic nervous system switches off the digestive processes, mobilizes stored sugar to the bloodstream and shifts the blood from our central core to the muscles of the limbs so that we can move quickly and save our life. It is designed for survival, but we cannot thrive in this state. Alas, most modern people live in this state.

With insufficient digestive enzymes, the food can feel like a brick in your stomach, stuck and not moving. Soon enough, in that warm and moist environment, it begins to ferment, producing gas so that the person feels bloated, uncomfortable and flatulent. The food starts to rot, and the toxins leach through the gut wall into the bloodstream, slightly poisoning the person so that they may develop headaches, feel mentally foggy and fatigued. The toxins may inflame the gut wall, causing gut permeability, so that large undigested food particles escape into the bloodstream where the patrolling immune cells come across them but don't recognize these large molecules as food and set up an immune response. In this way food intolerances are formed, as are autoimmune conditions, because sometimes the molecules look similar to our tissue cells, and so the immune system becomes confused and starts to attack both.

The fatigued and slightly poisoned person may reach for a sugary energy fix, which of course feeds the less helpful gut microbes such as yeasts, causing this population to explode, and the person to develop further yeast-related health problems.

There was a lot of sense when our grandparents insisted on sitting down at the table to eat in a convivial environment. Quite often, they took a digestive remedy which might have been a bitter-aromatic herbal liqueur to stimulate the digestive process. Further into this chapter is a recipe for a digestive tonic, but a quick and simple option is the tea below. Do not underestimate the importance of having your gut ready to receive and digest your food.

Another habit our grandparents adopted was to have a small sherry glass of pineapple juice before a heavier meal such as dinner. Pineapple contains a proteolytic enzyme called bromelain, which helps the hydrochloric acid break down and digest proteins such as meat and cheese. As we get older, our natural digestive enzymes decline, and so it can be helpful to support protein digestion by including proteolytic enzymes in our diets. Other proteolytic enzymes include papain, found in papaya, and actinidin from kiwi fruit.

## TEA TO AID DIGESTION
Make a mixture of the following herbs, and keep them dry, or simply add individual teabags to a teapot or mug of boiling water.

1 part ginger root
1 part peppermint leaves
1 part chamomile flowers
1 part fennel seeds

This may be drunk half an hour before or after food to relax the gut and encourage the secretion of digestive enzymes.

# SUPPORT YOUR FRIENDLY GUT POPULATION

Our friendly bacteria (known collectively as the microbiota, or biome) live not only in our intestines, but on every square millimetre of our bodies – even inside our lungs – and they perform many crucial functions in our body. We should think of them as a body system in their own right. When you consider that there are approximately 50 trillion cells in your body, and about 150 trillion bacteria within your body, it could be argued that we are more of a bacterial community than a single organism. Dead and alive bacteria make up 25 to 54 percent of the weight of the average adult stool, with approximately 100 billion bacteria per gram of wet stool.

So, you can imagine the disruption that happens when you take antibiotics, because these medicines kill not only the pathogenic bacteria causing illness, but also our natural bacterial biome.

The biome of our gut affects almost all aspects of human health. Healthy bacteria in your intestines help to metabolize and recycle the hormones, thereby helping to protect us from serious diseases like cancers. They also interact with our brain to affect our mood, cognition and pain perception. The biome maintains the integrity of our intestinal wall so that large undigested food molecules do not leak into the bloodstream causing autoimmune disease; it also converts nutrients, synthesizes vitamins and controls the growth of unfriendly bacteria and yeasts in our gut.[48]

We need to eat probiotic foods such as live plain yogurt, kefir, kimchi and fermented vegetables like sauerkraut and pickles to help reseed our gut with healthy bacteria.

Healthy organisms can also be found in the soil. If you are able to grow your own vegetables in organic soil, don't wash them too well. By eating them raw, you will be ingesting a wide variety of healthy bacteria which are extremely important in balancing your immune system as well as keeping a healthy digestive system.

The population of our gut varies according to the food we eat because certain bacteria feed on particular prebiotics (the foods from our diet which feed the microbiota), thus those following a vegetarian diet have a different population of microbiota to those following an omnivorous diet. We can help to promote a healthy population by eating probiotic foods, as well as plenty of fruit and vegetables, which are rich in prebiotics.

Prebiotic foods include apples, bananas, leeks, onions, garlic, Jerusalem artichokes, sweet potatoes, asparagus, barley and oats, potatoes and mushrooms.

# LIVER CONGESTION

Your liver is an amazing organ, performing over 500 functions which keep the exquisite homeostatic balances required for your body to function at all. With all the technology in the world today, there is still no machine that can perform the functions of this gland. It maintains our pH levels, breaks down and clears toxins from our body, stores blood and a form of readily available energy sugar, synthesizes proteins and stores fat-soluble vitamins, and regulates the balance of our sex hormones, as well as those of the thyroid and adrenal glands.

Amongst many functions of the liver, it also produces bile to emulsify dietary fat, allowing fat and fat-soluble vitamins to be absorbed into the blood. The bile itself is made up of bile salts and water, and with time, the bile salts can collect in the tiny tubules of the liver, congealing into bile sludge. This sludge can be easily seen by those who perform a liver/gallbladder flush (See *The Amazing Liver & Gallbladder Flush* by Andreas Moritz). The sludge can harden into grit and stones, which block up the liver, causing many health problems. Fortunately, our liver can be cleaned, and if necessary, it can regenerate (as can our heart, which recent evidence has shown).

You can significantly support your liver using simple kitchen remedies, then perhaps you may choose to progress onto Andreas Moritz's flush.

Apples contain malic acid which softens the stones and gravel in the liver. Grapefruit stimulates the bile flow, flushing out the softened sludge into the colon. If you simply eat one of each every day, you will go a long way toward keeping your liver in good health; however, there are other liver-supporting foods and culinary herbs for you to include in your diet.

## Household herbs and food which support liver function include:

🌿 **Rosemary** – antioxidant and liver protective

🌿 **Olive oil** – contains a substance called hydroxytyrosol, which has been shown to reverse the damage caused by a high-fat diet[49] [50]

🌿 **Ginger** – reduces cholesterol, has antioxidant effects and helps to reduce excessive blood sugars[51]

🌿 **Garlic** – antioxidants which protect against liver cancer and promote the clearing of free radicals

🌿 **Dandelion leaf and root** – both protect against fat accumulation and oxidative damage, reducing cholesterol levels and atherosclerosis (hardening and narrowing of the arteries)[52]

🌿 **Turmeric** – antioxidant, reduces scarring and thickening of the bile ducts and inflammation of the liver

🌿 **Globe artichoke leaf and heart** – antioxidative, protects against liver disease, encourages the flushing of bile, reduces cholesterol, has anti-obesity actions

🌿 **Apple cider vinegar** – reduces obesity, visceral and subcutaneous fat, protecting against metabolic syndrome[53]

🌿 **Hops** – inhibits several critical steps during the development of chronic liver disease, by blocking oxidative stress, inflammation, and hardening of the liver tissue[54]

🌿 **Beetroot (beets)** – protects against liver injury, is anti-inflammatory to the liver and removes toxins[55]

🌿 **Rocket (arugula) and chicory (endive)** – high chlorophyll helps to neutralize and detoxify the liver from heavy metals, and protect the cells from toxic damage; helps weight loss and reduces inflammation

🌿 **Brassica family** – supports healthy oestrogen balance by promoting the excretion of old hormones and shifting the balance toward protective oestrogens; in particular, raw vegetables, especially broccoli sprouts, are the most active in oestrogen clearing

🍃 **Radish** – powerful detoxifier of the liver, helps to flush old hormones from the body

🍃 **Lemon juice** – reverses alcoholic liver damage

🍃 **Grapefruit** – has anti-inflammatory effects on the liver, helping to clear fat build-up in the liver and reduce obesity

🍃 **Coffee** – reduces the risk of liver cancer, slows the rate of fibrosis in liver disease (fibrosis is the scar tissue build-up as a result of inflammation) and inhibits the development of cirrhosis[56]

A major cause of injury to the liver is oxidative damage, and when we review the therapeutic effects of these most well-known liver herbs, they almost all have powerful antioxidant properties. Nature is always ahead of the curve!

## LIVER TONIC
**To give your liver a morning flush, try this refreshing and warming liver tonic.**

5 slices of ginger
5 slices of fresh turmeric
1 slice of lemon
a sprig of rosemary

🍃 Add to a large mug of boiling water, allow to cool and drink 30 minutes before you eat breakfast.

# INCREASE YOUR FIBRE
Once the bile from your liver has flushed the waste into the colon, your dietary fibre (particularly seeds such as flaxseeds and chia) can grab onto waste matter by capturing the bile fluids within their surrounding mucilage. Chia or flaxseeds are particularly helpful for those who have hard dry stools because the mucilage which

surrounds the seeds absorbs the fluids in your large intestine, making the stool soft, slippery and easy to pass. The seed is said to "sweep the bowel", meaning that as it moves along the bowel, it gently brushes the sides of the colon, loosening and removing old faecal matter.

As the seeds expand, they gently stretch the colon, which stimulates natural bowel peristaltic movement. In this way, waste matter and liver toxins are safely and easily removed from your body.

## CONSTIPATION

Your bowel is designed to be stretched to a certain point by faecal matter, which will then trigger a peristaltic contraction in a wave-like motion, projecting the faecal matter in a clockwise direction out of the body. If our food lacks sufficient bulk in the form of vegetable fibre, that point of expansion followed by contraction occurs less frequently. The colon will continue to extract water from the faeces, resulting in dry hard pellets which are evacuated sporadically. The incomplete bowel movement leaves the person feeling bloated, and the toxins from the faeces are reabsorbed by the colon into the bloodstream, slowly poisoning the body. The result is that the person feels fatigued, suffers from bad breath and headaches. Often a sign of a sluggish bowel is a coated tongue. The trick is to increase your vegetable, fruit and salad intake.

The liver-cleansing programme below is an excellent remedy for constipation and does not involve senna or other stimulating laxatives. You will just find that when you go to the loo, you will have a large, easy and full bowel movement, leaving you feeling clean and fresh inside. This little programme can be followed at any time of the day, and is best done every day. The tea will help to stimulate bile flow, flushing toxins and bile sludge into the colon, where it is grabbed by the expanding seeds which will stimulate peristaltic movement, easily and efficiently eliminating the faecal matter. Of course, there are many delicious recipes which include flax or chia seeds, but the recipe below is one which I have given many times over the years, and is a firm favourite with my patients.

## A SIMPLE LIVER AND BOWEL DAILY CLEANSE

### PART 1: FLAX OR CHIA SEED YOGURT

120g (½ cup) of live, plain yogurt
2 tbsp freshly ground flaxseeds
    or chia seeds
a little fruit, if you wish

Immediately after eating the yogurt, drink the herbal tea when cool enough.

### PART 2: LIVER-FLUSH TEA

1 tsp apple cider vinegar
1 slice of lemon
a sprig of mint
1 large mug of boiling water

# INDIGESTION

Dyspepsia or indigestion is a common problem and one caused either by our ageing and declining digestive enzymes or by stress. You can feel as if you have a stone in your stomach, because you cannot digest your food, and often, there is also acid reflux. It may seem strange but over-acidity and under-acidity have the same symptoms. One way to test is to have an apple cider tea after food, and if your symptoms improve then you have too little acid and the following advice will help you.

Fruits are rich in enzymes which can help you to digest your food, but there are three fruits particularly rich in proteolytic (protein-digesting) enzymes, and these are fresh pineapple, kiwi fruit and papaya. You can test this by placing a slice of ham on a fresh pineapple slice. Within hours the ham will turn to pate. You must use fresh pineapple or papaya, because the enzymes are destroyed in the cooking process, so canned pineapple will not help you.

Herbalists have used bitter herbs for hundreds of years to improve digestion by stimulating the flow of bile and digestive enzymes. This is appropriate for older or very unwell people. For younger people, the problem is usually related to stress, and then we use relaxing bitter herbs like hops and vervain.

A cup of chamomile tea or catnip tea helps to relax the digestive tract, and is especially valuable for the upset child. Hops is a stronger herb. Like chamomile, it is calming and both have the bitter principles which stimulate the digestive enzymes to flow.

Herbs with bitter principles have been appreciated since at least the medieval era. The famous medieval German abbess Hildegard von Bingen was a most excellent herbalist, and she created a bitter tonic formula which is said to still be used today to improve digestion and reduce the cravings for sugar. Not all the herbs are available to the lay person, but many are. Herbs such as wormwood, bitter oranges, ginger, cardamom, turmeric, dandelion root, yarrow, angelica root, fennel, lavender and cumin seeds formed a significant part of her bitter tonic. It could be a fun project to collect these herbs and steep them in gin or sweet wine to take as an after-dinner liqueur.

## AFTER-DINNER LIQUEUR

10g (⅓oz) fennel seeds

10g (⅓oz) chopped and dried
   orange peel

10g (⅓oz) dried ginger root

10g (⅓oz) chamomile flowers

10g (⅓oz) peppermint leaves

10g (⅓oz) angelica root (grow and
   harvest yourself, or purchase
   from a herbalist)

10g (⅓oz) dried and crushed
   hops cones

10g (⅓oz) caraway seeds

🌿 The herbs can be added to a sweetish wine or gin (750ml), and allowed to steep for about a month before straining and bottling. A small sherry glass can be taken before or after a meal.

🌿 If you prefer, you can use the herbs as an infusion instead. Steep 1 teaspoon of herbs per cup of boiling water, making sure to cover the teapot so that you preserve the essential oils which rise with the steam. Drink after a meal to promote comfortable digestion.

~~~~~~~~~~~~~~~~~~~~~~~~~~

# STOMACH CRAMPS

If you regularly suffer from stomach cramps, you really must see a doctor, especially if you find blood or mucus in your stool. If mainstream medicine doesn't find anything with their tests, then consider a nutritionist or medical herbalist. Having said that, we all know that stress frequently manifests as tummy cramps. I have seen this so often with children, who don't really understand that they are anxious, but they do know that their tummy hurts. Adults who are still locked in with childhood anxieties like excessive shyness or dealing with a scary teacher (now an overbearing boss) can suffer from irritable bowel syndrome. It is as if the intestines can tell us what the head doesn't want to admit.

Another reason may be a parasite infection, which needs to be addressed. You might clearly remember diarrhoea on a foreign holiday, or vomiting after a meal, and having never felt quite right after that. Parasites really require professional support, so I shan't elaborate further on that subject.

Gas and bloating can also cause cramping. The underlying causes here may be a yeast overgrowth, too much sugar in the diet, wheat or lactose intolerance, poor digestion, constipation or parasites.

If you suffer from persistent cramps, please do get it checked, but if you rarely have this problem then there are a few herbal teas which can give much relief.

Peppermint, fennel and ginger are excellent options and easy to come by. When people call me with tummy cramps and I am away, and therefore unable to send stronger herbs, I usually suggest some simple teas (to follow).

## Hops (*Humulus lupulus*)

Hops is my favourite herb to use with irritable bowels. The green cones should be harvested at the end of summer, and the lovely spicy fragrance fills the home as you dry them for your winter decorations or sleep pillows.

Hops are deeply relaxing herbs, and also have a bitterness to them, making them absolutely perfect for people who are anxious with a seized-up gut, flatulence and poor digestion. One cone goes a long way, and do be aware that hops can make you sleepy, so it is worth using this herb sparingly. Once the hops are dried, you can crush them so that the petals separate.

## Lavender (*Lavendula angustifolia*)

Lavender is not a herb often associated with the digestive tract, but it is a relaxing herb, and aromatic, which means that it stimulates the digestive juices to flow as the smells from the kitchen do. I find it particularly useful for the anxious gut, and it may be used with, or instead of, hops or chamomile. Use it sparingly because it has a strong fragrance and you don't want an overpowering flavour. The idea is to gently bring the stomach back to a comfortable condition.

Lavender will make a person less sleepy than hops, so it is more of a daytime herb, whereas hops is more of a night-time herb. Having said that, when I am treating irritable bowel syndrome I always include a tiny bit of hops, and nobody falls asleep at their desk. They just feel so much more comfortable in their digestive tract, and within themselves.

**Other herbs to relax the gut include:**

- Chamomile flowers
- Fennel seeds
- Peppermint leaves
- Ginger root
- Caraway seeds
- Catnip

## EMERGENCY TEA FOR STOMACH CRAMPS

1 peppermint teabag
1 fennel teabag
1 chamomile teabag
5 slices of fresh ginger

Brew the herbs in a mug of boiling water until cool enough to drink.

## EVENING DIGESTIVE TEA

a pinch of hops cone petals
1 chamomile tea bag
1 fennel or mint tea bag
1 head of dried or fresh lavender

Drop all of these into a teapot, cover with boiling water and steep until cool enough to drink. This can be taken after a meal to settle the stomach, and give you a lovely peaceful sleep.

## TUMMY TEA FOR CHILDREN

1 chamomile tea bag
1 fennel seed tea bag
1 sprig of catnip

Pop these into a small teapot, cover with boiling water and allow to cool. Add a little honey to taste, and let the child sip this in a comfortable environment.

# GASTRITIS AND GASTRIC ULCERS

Gastritis causes symptoms of nausea, gnawing hunger pains and burning under the breastbone. Bleeding ulcers can cause these symptoms as well as black blood in the stool. The hydrochloric acid in our stomach is tremendously corrosive, and designed for breaking down tough meat fibres. It is a miracle that when we eat, our stomachs are not digested too. However, when one has an ulcer or gastritis, that is partially what has happened because the protective lining of the stomach has been eroded, and the acid is burning the wall of the stomach. It is important that a protective lining is immediately restored, and the gut wall is healed as quickly as possible.

The underlying cause of the gastritis or ulcer must be addressed too. It is frequently caused by a bacterium called *Helicobacter pylori*, or by the excessive use of non-steroidal anti-inflammatory medicines for pain. These two causes must be addressed by a professional, but until then, you can at least protect your stomach lining from further damage.

The old approach is to adopt a bland diet. Whilst this has fallen out of fashion, there is a lot of sense in it, in that it keeps the flow of digestive juices to a minimum. Foods like well-cooked vegetables, white rice, mashed potato and poached white fish sound very unexciting, but that is the idea. We do not want to excite the stomach into secreting too much acid until the corrosion has been healed.

# Slippery elm or marshmallow and aloe vera

Slippery elm, marshmallow and aloe vera (or aloe ferox) are all demulcent herbs. This means that they are slippery and soothing, coating the gut lining and protecting it from the hydrochloric acid. The slippery elm and marshmallow can be used interchangeably, but I prefer marshmallow root, because it is locally sourced and sustainable. Slippery elm is the bark of a tree, whilst marshmallows are easily grown shrubs and thus very environmentally friendly.

When using aloe, make sure that you use the filleted leaf and not whole-leaf extract. The healing constituents are found in the inner sap, whilst the outer leaf has a laxative effect. At this time, you need the healing actions. Aloe vera or ferox are tremendously healing to the underlying tissues of the stomach. Taking slippery elm or marshmallow with aloe will both protect the gut and stimulate the healing of the damaged cells.

Adding a little turmeric powder also reduces the pain and stimulates the healing of the damaged tissues.

## HEALING MILK FOR GASTRIC EROSIONS

1 heaped tsp slippery elm powder
    or marshmallow root powder
4 tsp aloe vera inner leaf juice
    (do not use whole leaf juice)

🌿 Whisk these ingredients into a glass of dairy or vegetable milk, then drink. Or, if you prefer, add to a little warm dairy or vegetable milk to eat as a porridge.

🌿 Do this 3 times a day between meals and you will feel immediate relief. As this is very safe, you can take this drink up to 5 times a day.

## Cabbage juice

Older generations used to drink cabbage water to heal their stomach linings. This was the water left over from the boiling of cabbage as a vegetable. These days, raw cabbage juice is advocated for its healing due to vitamin U. Very few studies have been done on the effect of cabbage on peptic ulcers, but one from 1949 shows that it healed gastric ulcers up to four times more quickly than without the use of cabbage juice.[57] To make cabbage juice, simply run a cabbage through the juicer and divide the dose, drinking a quarter of the juice on an empty stomach four times a day.

## Butter

Organic, grass-fed butter is rich in a substance known as butyric acid, which provides a beneficial food for the cells of the gut. It is a natural anti-inflammatory and helps to regulate the peristaltic movements of the bowel, and can also help to prevent colonic cancer. There are farms which sell butter from cows who are allowed to keep their calves with them until naturally weaned, rather than having them taken away after one day or seven days, as is the case of non-organic and organic butter respectively. The butter is more expensive, but you are paying for a natural process with a calm and contented cow. Her immune system is not depleted by the stress and grief, the butter rich and delicious. You can taste the contentment and kindness.

## Bone broth and gelatine

For those with a really raw and sore tummy, bone broth is a safe and easily absorbable source of nutrients, especially for those needing to heal an inflamed and leaky gut. Rich in glutamine and collagen, it provides the stomach and intestines with the nutrients needed to rebuild the gut walls, and repair the damage caused by the inflammation. Bone broth can be made from beef, lamb, chicken or fish bones, and vegetables. To make it even more healing, you might like to add a little extra gelatine (collagen), turmeric (anti-inflammatory) and some healthy butter (food for the intestinal cells).

## CABBAGE AND BONE BROTH

🌿 Finely slice a savoy cabbage, and poach in bone broth until very soft.

🌿 When all is cooked, add a good dollop of butter and eat as a broth.

# DIGESTIVE SHUT-DOWN

When people have been unwell, their digestive tract can shut down, and they lose the inclination to eat. The elderly are often in this position too, and they love to eat soft, sweet foods like desserts and yogurts because they are easy to digest and the sugar gives them a little boost. When the digestive system is partially shut down, the enzymes are not available to digest the food, and again, the meal is stuck in the gut, fermenting and causing nausea and discomfort. And yet, in order to recover from an illness, the person needs nutritious foods.

Both the elderly and the very ill cannot cope with large portions of foods, and indeed a full plate can be very off-putting. Tiny portions more often and nourishing soups are more in line with what the gut can cope with. My mother was once very close to death with a viral infection and antibiotic poisoning. Her digestive system had shut down and the thought of food made her nauseous. When I arrived to help her, we started with a small square of avocado pear, a grape and a teaspoon of cottage cheese. Later, she had a little creamed spinach and a soft-boiled egg, and later again a little bone-broth soup. The idea is to tempt the gut with tiny portions of easily digestible, very nourishing foods, and the patient will ask for more food as they are able to cope with it.

In order to reawaken the digestive tract, warming aromatic herbs like ginger, fresh turmeric and fennel can gently stimulate the intestines to secrete the enzymes.

Infusions are the most appropriate for weak digestive systems, because alcohol is far too harsh, and they just cannot digest tablets or capsules. The infusion is easily absorbed and soothing on the stomach lining. This tea is particularly helpful for those who feel "cold" in their stomach. It is helpful for the elderly and those who are very unwell. By warming and relaxing the stomach, it is happier to receive and digest food.

## TEA TO REAWAKEN THE DIGESTIVE PROCESS

2 slices of ginger

1 peppermint tea bag

1 chamomile tea bag

a sprig of lemon balm or catnip

1 slice of lemon

a little honey to taste

🌿 Put all the herbs into a thermos flask with boiling water, and pour out just a little every hour for the person to take.

## TRAVELLER'S STOMACH

It is one of the least charming aspects of travelling to exotic and far-flung destinations. Delhi Belly, Pharaoh's Revenge, call it what you may, traveller's gastritis and diarrhoea can be devastating to your holiday plans, and once nearly killed me. But that was back in those days when I was a backpacking kid, and I didn't know what to do. Now I do, and I give all my travelling patients these tips, and they are usually the only ones who come back without incident – from their guts, anyway.

🌿 The first step is to take enough *Saccharomyces boulardii* for the duration of your trip, and 1 week afterwards. You will need a capsule which contains 5 billion probiotic yeasts every day, plus extra capsules in case you do catch a stomach bug.

🌿 Bring with you a whole bulb of raw garlic.

🌿 And some powdered cinnamon.

🌿 Each day, after breakfast, you take 1 capsule of *S. boulardii*. The probiotic yeast is the natural enemy of bad bacteria and crowds out any nasty bugs.

🌿 Before bed, you chop up 1 clove of garlic and swallow it with a drink. For a few minutes, you may feel quite nauseous and think that you are going to vomit, but you won't. The feeling passes rapidly. The garlic kills the pathogenic bacteria which might have got into your gut. During the night you will breathe off any offending odours.

🌿 If you do catch a tummy bug, taking anti-diarrhoea medications is not necessarily the best approach, because the medicines simply paralyse your gut, which stops the diarrhoea but also traps the bacteria in your body. Diarrhoea is a natural mechanism designed to evict harmful bacteria from your gut. You need to kill the bacteria and get it out of your body. This is what you can do, and if you are not better within two days, do see a doctor.

## SOME POSITIVE TIPS IF YOU DO CATCH A TUMMY BUG.

🌿 Take a crushed garlic clove morning and evening *before* your meal (if, indeed you can face food), and an *S. bourlardii* capsule morning and evening *after* your meal. If you can't bear the garlic, then just take the *S. bourlardii*, but do try the garlic as it is very helpful.

🌿 Add ½ teaspoon of cinnamon powder to a cup of boiling water and sip. This will help to kill the invading bugs, whilst helping to settle your stomach.

🌿 Don't forget to rehydrate with electrolyte drinks.

# YEAST AND FUNGAL INFECTIONS

When antibiotics have been taken orally, they massively disrupt the populations of the gut, killing off the pathogenic bacteria as well as the friendly bacterial population, but not the yeast which also live in your gut. As such, yeast populations such as candida explode when the gut bacteria are not there to restrict their growth. Think of a mushroom popping up overnight on an autumnal lawn, or bread dough rising. The fungi are very opportunistic.

Add to this scenario the Western diet, which is very high in sugar, and the yeasts are in heaven. Your gut is a lovely dark, moist and sweet environment without any enemies – and it is party time for candida.

Common symptoms of yeast overgrowth include oral, vaginal or anal thrush (an itchy bottom); brain fog with difficulty focussing and sometimes even difficulty holding a conversation; mood disturbances; a bloated and flatulent digestive system; irritable bowel syndrome; yeast infections of the skin; ongoing fatigue; aching joints. This condition needs professional attention, but if you have to take antibiotics, you can nip the overgrowth in the bud with some simple remedies.

The most important thing you must do is repopulate your gut with friendly bacteria. Take a good probiotic, drink kefir and eat some live sauerkraut. These foods seed your gut with the friendly bacteria. Then you feed the friendly bacteria with plenty of vegetables which contain prebiotics such as fructo-oligosaccharides (FOS) and inulin. All vegetables contain prebiotics, so just make sure that you have a healthy and varied diet. Of course, you completely stop all sugar, and for a while, give up bread, pasta and other stodgy foods which break down into sugar in the gut, and alcohol. Finally, you kill.

You can use plants to push the yeast back into its small population numbers within your gut. Remember that we don't completely kill it off, because you can't, and because it has a function. We will never know everything about life, and there is some evidence that candida helps to detoxify mercury from our bodies.

The probiotic bacteria can crowd out the yeast overgrowth, but sometimes you need to take stronger action. There are some herbs and spices in your kitchen cupboard and on your windowsill, which are a really good start. If you need to use stronger supplements and herbs, I strongly suggest that you see a medical herbalist, nutritionist or naturopath because treating candida is a complicated business, and if you get it wrong, you can make things worse for yourself.

If you have had antibiotics, are feeling uncomfortable in your gut, and thrush has flared, try this tea using a common and lovely house plant. Rose geranium is powerfully antifungal, calming, and makes a delicious tea.

## ANTI-YEAST TEA

2 leaves of rose geranium – if you don't have rose geranium, add ½ tsp of kitchen dried thyme (these herbs can be alternated each day)
½ tsp cinnamon powder
1 clove

🌿 Drop these ingredients into a teapot and add a cup of boiling water. Quickly cover with the lid, and drink when cooled.

🌿 Drink 3 cups of this tea per day for 5 days. If the yeast infection does not clear up, please see your medical herbalist or naturopathic practitioner.

*If you have had antibiotics, are feeling uncomfortable in your gut, and thrush has flared, try this tea using a common and lovely house plant.*

## Raw garlic

Garlic is also powerfully antifungal, so include plenty of raw garlic in your food. Cooked garlic isn't strong enough – you need the smelly elements.

A really simple way to take garlic is to crush a clove of organic garlic. Leave it for five minutes and then swallow with a vegetable or dairy milk. You may feel nauseous for a few minutes as if you are going to vomit, but you won't. Just lie down for a minute or two, and then you can get on with your life. This is best done at night before bed, as your body will have time to breathe off the odours, and you are less likely to be whiffy the next day. In the morning, you can take a probiotic after breakfast.

### GARLIC TOAST

Toast some coarse German rye bread. Rub both sides with raw garlic.

Spread with avocado pear or sliced tomatoes and drizzle with olive oil.

### Other antifungal kitchen herbs include:

Cinnamon

Oregano

Thyme

Include these generously in your cooking, and most important of all: give up sugar.

## Give up sugar

Ours is a high-speed lifestyle, frequently fuelled by caffeine and sugar, but it is not sustainable, except for the yeasts that thrive in this environment. One of the most important ways to support your health is through your diet, and giving up sugar, alcohol and refined stodgy carbohydrates. This can be very difficult because our culture is addicted to sugar and wine.

A sugar hit makes you feel fantastic – you can take on the world! Then your insulin packs the sugar away into your fat cells, your blood sugar levels plummet, and you feel awful. You may reach for the coffee, and maybe a biscuit to keep you going, and so it goes on – a yoyo diet which is absolutely exhausting for our bodies.

When you give up sugar, and those foods which turn into sugar – like alcohol and bread or pasta – you starve the yeast and their population starts to shrink back. You will also find yourself snacking on more healthy foods, like a hard-boiled egg, avocado, raw nuts or vegetables and hummus.

This change of diet, with food-state probiotics such as kefir, sauerkraut, kimchi, kombucha or pickles, and the antifungal tea on page 173, should leave you feeling much better. If you don't feel well within three weeks, I do urge you to see a naturopathic practitioner such as a medical herbalist or nutritionist.

When I am treating long-term candida, it is sometimes painful for my patients to hear that they cannot have any sugar at all. No fruit either. Happily, these days we have a get-out-of-jail-free option in the form of stevia or xylitol. Both of these natural sweeteners are fine to use in moderation if you have candida, as a little treat. Overleaf are four small desserts that you can enjoy from time to time.

## MUHALLABIA

This is a variation on a delicious Middle Eastern dessert. Enhance the Arabian-nights theme by serving with a small glass of mint tea.

½ cup of almond yogurt
1 tsp rose water, or orange
    blossom water
a sprinkle of stevia or xylitol
seeds from 1 cardamom pod
a few pistachio nuts
rose petals (optional)

🌿 Combine the yogurt, rose or orange blossom water and sweetener in a bowl and set aside.

🌿 Drop the cardamom seeds and pistachios into a hot dry pan to release the fragrances. Toss the seeds and nuts about so as not to let them burn, then put into a mortar and pestle and crush.

🌿 Sprinkle over the top of your dessert, and you might like to add a few small and fragrant fresh rose petals.

## TURKISH DELIGHT ANTIFUNGAL PUDDING

2 squares of 90% dark chocolate
1 level tbsp mascarpone cheese
1 tsp stevia
1 drop of rose geranium essential oil

🌿 Melt together the chocolate, mascarpone and sweetener in a bain-marie.

🌿 Once the cheese/chocolate has melted, add the rose geranium essential oil, mix well, and pour into a ramekin dish.

🌿 Allow to cool and enjoy in moderation.

## SUGAR-FREE MOCHA DESSERT

2 squares of 90% dark chocolate
1 level tbsp mascarpone cheese
1 tsp stevia
4 tsp strong coffee
double (heavy) cream

🌿 Melt together the chocolate, mascarpone and sweetener in a bain-marie. Then add the coffee.

🌿 Cream all the ingredients together, then pour into a sherry glass so that it is two-thirds full. Place in the refrigerator.

🌿 When chilled, pour cream over the top, so that it looks like an Irish coffee.

## BLUEBERRY 'PANCAKE' FOR AFTERNOON TEA

🌿 Whisk 2 eggs and 1 tablespoon of wheatgerm together.

🌿 Pour into a lightly oiled frying pan to cook as an omelette.

🌿 Quickly toss in a small handful of fresh blueberries and allow the omelette to cook.

🌿 By the time the egg has coagulated, the blueberries will have broken down into blue/black pools of jammy fruitiness.

🌿 Now sprinkle with some cinnamon powder and a little xylitol if you wish.

🌿 Fold over in half and serve on a plate.

# Carob

A really fabulous non-sugary option is carob. This is a Mediterranean food, derived from the pods of the carob tree (*Ceratonia siliqua*). Also known as the locust bean, these pods were probably the "locusts" that John the Baptist lived on. The pod itself is quite delicious, and I love to chew on one when I am on Mediterranean land. I once found some horses and, thinking I was being kind, I gave a horse one to enjoy. He loved it, so I collected more, and gave each of the horses in their stables a treat. Well, it all got a bit scary, because they were so excited that they nearly jumped out of their stables, and I quickly threw the pods down and beat a sheepish and hasty retreat.

Apart from being really tasty, they are also rich in vitamins and minerals, including vitamin A and some B vitamins, iron, calcium, magnesium, potassium, zinc and selenium. They also contain lots of antioxidants, and are high in fibre and tannins.

Processed carob looks like chocolate but doesn't taste like chocolate. It has a soft malty sweetness and – this is what we are interested in – it has a low glycaemic index.

Although carob tastes sweet, it has been shown to significantly lower blood sugar and cholesterol levels. With its high fibre content, it keeps the stomach fuller for longer, but more than that, it decreases ghrelin, the hormone which makes us hungry. Rabbits fed with carob in their food lost weight.

For conditions like candida and diabetes, carob can be invaluable, both in providing for a sweet tooth, but also by helping to reduce blood sugar levels. Intestinal candida can inflame and damage the gut, and here, carob may be helpful too because traditionally carob has been used to treat diarrhoea and is so gentle that it may even be used for babies. I love to use it for very tender and inflamed digestive tracts, especially when combined with slippery elm and marshmallow root. It makes a soothing, nourishing, healing convalescence food for those with gastritis, candida and colitis.

Opposite are three of my favourite luscious carob recipes.

## SLIPPERY PORRIDGE FOR VERY SORE AND INFLAMED DIGESTIVE TRACTS

2 tbsp slippery elm powder
1 tbsp carob powder
¾ cup of oat milk

🍃 Mix the powders with cold or warm oat milk until a smooth porridge is achieved.

🍃 Eat little and often.

## HOT CAROB DRINK FOR BLOOD-SUGAR CONTROL

1 cup of oat milk (high fibre regulates blood sugar levels)
2 tsp carob powder (for sweetness but reduces blood sugar levels)
⅓ tsp cinnamon powder (antifungal, reduces blood sugar levels)

🍃 Warm the oat milk gently in a saucepan. Whisk in the carob and cinnamon and drink.

## CAROB SUPERFOOD TREAT

🍃 Place a saucepan in a frying pan of hot water, then add a large tablespoon of coconut oil. Add sufficient carob powder so that the powder is absorbed by the coconut oil. Keep adding until the oil cannot absorb any more carob powder.

🍃 Pour this sludge onto a piece of greaseproof (waxed) paper, and pat it into a thinnish layer. Quickly sprinkle with both roughly and finely chopped walnuts and goji berries, slightly patting them down so that they are embedded in the carob.

🍃 When it has cooled, you can snap it into small pieces to snack on. The nuts provide good-quality omega oils and slow the absorption of the sugar. The goji berries provide a lovely sweet/sharp toffeeness, but are highly antioxidant and super healthy.

I do emphasize seeing a professional nutritionist or medical herbalist, and there is a sound reason for this. When you kill candida (or other pathogens or parasites), the dead organisms break down and release their toxins into the bloodstream, which can make you feel really ill if your liver has not been prepared. This is called a Herxheimer reaction, or die-off. A medical herbalist or naturopath will prepare your liver, consider why you have the yeast overgrowth, or the original illness which may have caused you to need the antibiotics, and treat the underlying causes of the illness. In other words, candida is just the tip of an iceberg which really does need professional help. However, if you are normally very well, have had to take antibiotics, and now have thrush or a funny tummy, the above will help you and you should make a full recovery.

Taking into account all the information in the chapter, below is a recipe to use every day to support a healthy digestive system.

## MORNING SMOOTHIE
## FOR A HEALTHY DIGESTIVE SYSTEM

2 tbsp chia seeds (bowel sweep)

a handful of blackberries, blueberries or raspberries (antioxidants)

some fresh pineapple or papaya (digestive enzymes)

a handful of kale (gut-wall healing, but leave out if you are hypothyroid)

2 stalks of fresh celery (liver cleansing)

a small handful of fresh mint (normalizes peristaltic movement)

a good dollop of live plain dairy or vegan yogurt, or kefir (probiotics)

vegetable milk of your choice, or plain water

Whizz everything together to make a smoothie.

I like to make this the night before. The chia seeds make this a very soothing drink, and the whole smoothie helps to cleanse your colon gently and effectively.

# BABY COLIC

Finally, we come to our little people, who can suffer greatly from what I have called "screaming colic". Many is the time when I have helped a baby find relief within minutes by giving them drops from the following recipe.

## COLIC DROPS

If your baby develops colic, you can either dip your finger a few times in a little of this colic glycerite, and allow the infant to suck; otherwise, add a teaspoon to their bottle, which keeps their tummies comfortable. The baby will settle very quickly.

3 tsp fennel seeds
3 tsp fresh German chamomile flowers
2 tsp fresh catnip
100ml (3½fl oz) vegetable glycerine

🌿 Place the herbs in a teapot, and cover with 100ml (3½fl oz) boiling water. Quickly pop the lid on and leave until cool.

🌿 Carefully strain through a muslin-lined sieve into a funnel and into a bottle.

🌿 Add the vegetable glycerine. Shake, seal and label.

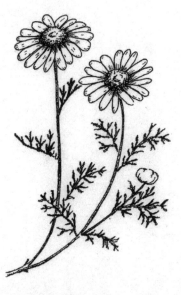

# CHAPTER 7

## Autumn Equinox

Late September is a beautiful time of year, and for many in the northern hemisphere, autumn is their favourite season. The air is still warm, berries festoon the hedgerows, and golden leaves flash and skitter as they fall from the trees. It is a time of nostalgia, when we hold onto the memory of frolicking on warm summer days, whilst we anticipate with some dread (or relief) the frosty cold soon to come, yet we also relish the idea of being snug in our homes, enjoying hearty meals shared with family and friends. Perhaps the bounty of the harvest makes us think of those less fortunate than us, or those in need, for the season of harvest may remind us to share some of our bounty. What is the point of money if we can't use it to help our fellow wayfarers treading this beautiful Earth? The balance of life is never fairly tipped toward equality.

Although the strength of the sun has long started to wane, at this time of equal dark and light, we can no longer ignore the fact that we have to prepare for the change of season, both in our outer world and also our inner world. If we allow ourselves to follow cycles of nature, we will naturally slow down and quieten down, starting to turn reflectively inward, as, at the same time, we gently prepare for the year ahead. In this, we are reminded of the goddess Persephone, who was seized by Hades and taken to live in the underworld for part of the year. Persephone was the Greek goddess of vegetation, and she represents the grains sown by the farmers. The seeds live in the underworld for the winter months before re-emerging as verdant spring crops.

Now, at this time of balance, just at the tipping point of the seasons, we may reflect upon the little seasons and the greater seasons of our own body, so often governed by the balance of hormones. Women are almost always aware of their hormonal cycles, both monthly and as we age. The balance shifts for men too from their mid-forties, as the andropause starts to take effect. Sometimes the changes can bring unwanted symptoms, and once again, we turn to the benevolent power of plants to restore balance to the turbulence of our own changing seasons.

# YOUR HORMONAL BALANCE

🍂 MUGWORT 🍂 VERVAIN 🍂 ROSE GERANIUM 🍂 CLIVERS
🍂 WILLOW HERB 🍂 HORSETAIL 🍂 NETTLE ROOT

It may seem slightly off-piste to say that your hormonal balance has a great deal to do with the state of your liver and colon. If your organs of elimination are congested, then the hormones cannot be metabolized and excreted, which leads to associated symptoms such as headaches, fatigue, anger and tearfulness, cold hands and feet, bloating and breast engorgement. Before we even consider herbs to support your hormones, you must pay attention to your liver and colon. You will find this information in Chapter 6.

A great many health irregularities can be normalized by a healthy diet – food being your primary medicine – and by using old-fashioned naturopathic techniques such as liver cleansing. Cutting out wheat, sugar and dairy products, and increasing vegetables, salads and fruit, grains, pulses, nuts and seeds, a few eggs, and a little organic meat and fish will lighten your system and allow the body to function optimally. Grapefruit is particularly helpful in supporting the liver to decongest.

Working on the assumption that you have read Chapter 6, and paid attention to your liver and digestive system, we can now turn our attention to your hormones.

## PRE-MENSTRUAL SYNDROME

For some women, up to a third of their month can be dominated by the difficult symptoms of premenstrual syndrome. That does not make for a comfortable life, but fortunately, plants can be extremely effective in restoring balance to the hormones. Strangely enough, there is little clear understanding as to the causes of PMS, but if you look at the menstrual cycle chart, you can plainly see that just before menstruation, both oestrogen and progesterone levels, and sometimes serotonin, drops. Small wonder some women feel low and tearful. It is also a time when many women feel extra sensitive, and often wish to spend time alone. If you are able to find time to be on your own, this can be a beautiful period when you connect with your inner peace through meditation or reflection.

The safest and cleverest of all the hormonal herbs is *Vitex agnus-castus*, which balances our hormones from the level of the pituitary gland. Somehow, this herb seems to know just what to do, and quite often, simply using agnus castus is enough to balance the hormones. Combining agnus castus with a good-quality evening primrose oil supplement (up to 1,500mg daily) is often all that is needed to balance the hormones and restore tranquillity to your life.

My experience is that women who feel tearful and crave chocolate respond very well to plants like red clover or sage, which gently top up the oestrogen levels, while women who feel angry, bloated and whose skin is affected often do better with the liver herbs such as mugwort.

## Mugwort (*Artemisia vulgaris*)

Around a thousand years ago, a herbal document called the *Lacnunga* gave reverential tribute to a herb they called "Una", the most ancient of all the herbs. Today we call her mugwort. Her botanical name (*Artemisia vulgaris*) is after Artemis, the Greek goddess of the moon and protector of women's health.

These days, mugwort is barely noticed as she grows alongside the motorway and in unused places – a beautiful and powerful goddess standing proudly amongst the filth of the city. But she is still precious to women, and those who use dreams to access the subconscious.

Herbalists use mugwort for many reasons, particularly for indigestion, intestinal parasites and pre-menstrual syndrome.

The herb is bitter, yet pleasant to drink as a tea, and it helps to decongest the liver. Very little of this herb is needed to alleviate the pre-menstrual symptoms of bloating, breast engorgement and irrational anger, so that the woman feels so much lighter in her body and her mood; she is calmer and more patient, with her period arriving easily, the whole cycle smoothed out. Mugwort can bring on heavier periods, so if your periods are already heavy, this may not be the herb for you.

**CAUTION:** This is not a herb to take if you are pregnant as it is a stimulant to the uterus and can cause abortion.

## Vervain (*Verbena officinalis*)
Vervain is another treasure for PMS, and like mugwort, is easily grown in your garden or allotment. It is slightly bitter, which means that it cleanses the liver, supports oestrogen levels and is a calming herb. Herbalists say that it is as comforting as a mother's hug, and when I prescribe it for pre-menstrual syndrome, women tell me that they move from being an upset, irrational person to feeling "normal again", which is a great relief.

## Rose geranium (*Pelargonium graveolens*)
Rose geranium is a common essential oil, but it is also a common house plant which people forget may be used as a herbal tea. It is indigenous to South Africa, where it is sometimes enjoyed in milk desserts, and it does make a most delicious tea which balances the hormones and calms the nerves.

A recent study showed rose geranium to be antidepressant, alleviate anxiety and to cleanse the lymphatic system, amongst many other benefits, thus it would clearly be of benefit for those suffering from pre-menstrual syndrome.[58] Another study showed that simply the inhalation of rose geranium was able to upregulate oestrogen levels in women who were peri-menopausal.[59] Because pre-menstrual symptoms and symptoms of peri-menopause are related to a drop of hormonal levels, it is clear why rose geranium can help to alleviate these distressing symptoms.

## ESSENTIAL OILS

Essential oils can also help with pre-menstrual syndrome. Lemon or grapefruit are bright, sunny and joyful essential oils which encourage the liver to secrete bile when inhaled. When you flush bile, the toxins stuck in the liver cells are also washed out of that organ. Lavender and clary sage are both deeply relaxing essential oils, and have an anti-spasmodic effect on the muscles.

Rose and rose geranium bring a sense of peace and balance, reducing depression, especially effective for women. Both are said to balance the female hormonal system, but I could not find many studies to support this; however, countless aromatherapists have attested to this effect, which I think is evidence enough. I once saw a very agitated mare in season, snapping and kicking at the other horses in the stables. When rosewater was vaporized into her stable, she immediately calmed down. With animals, the argument for placebo doesn't hold.

## ESSENTIAL OIL BLEND
## TO BALANCE THE HORMONES

This blend of essential oils can be used in a vaporizer, or dropped on a blank inhaler or even a tissue and left on your desk so that you inhale the aroma all day.

1 drop of lemon or grapefruit
2 drops of high-altitude lavender
3 drops of rose geranium
1 drop of clary sage

*Rose and rose geranium bring a sense of peace and balance, reducing depression, especially effective for women.*

# BREAST ENGORGEMENT AND LUMPS

Once again, it is very important to support the liver's function of metabolizing and clearing the accumulation of hormones, but it is also important to pay attention to the lymphatic system, as the lymph nodes in the breast tissue often become congested. One of the herbs that I find fabulous for this condition is clivers. It is very safe and has a cleansing effect on the entire glandular and lymphatic system. The other supplements which are fabulous for breast congestion include evening primrose oil and *Vitex agnus-castus*, both best taken in the morning before food.

## Clivers/goosegrass/sticky willy (*Galium aparine*)

During the early summer months, *Galium* is easily taken by simply pulling a handful out of the hedge, rolling it up and pushing it into a glass of water. Leave overnight and drink this every morning. To continue to use it throughout the year, you need to collect the herb, crush it and macerate it in apple cider vinegar. I even whizz the vinegar and the herb in my food processor, leave it overnight and then press it through muslin. This will keep in the refrigerator for months, and can be taken as a tablespoon every day in a glass of water.

# PERIOD PAIN

Period pain can either occur before the actual menstruation or as the menstruation begins, continuing for a few days. They have separate causes, but are quite easily differentiated, although some women suffer from both types of pain.

Congestive pre-menstrual pain often begins before the menstruation, usually followed by thick clotty bleeding – this is caused by sluggish pelvic circulation. This is the type of period pain where you feel swollen, bloated and irritable, as if you want to burst, and it is a great relief when the bleeding begins. The pain is quite often simply remedied by ginger, and if you have some, yarrow (*Achillea millefolium*). You can make a tea with fresh ginger and yarrow, and drink this daily for one week before your period to improve the pelvic circulation. You will find very quickly that your menstrual blood is bright and red, and that you feel far more comfortable.

The other type of period pain is caused by cramping. There are herbs which are very helpful but they should be carefully considered by a medical herbalist; however, ginger comes to the rescue once again as a warming anti-spasmodic herb. Non-steroidal anti-inflammatories such as ibuprofen are often prescribed because they block the release of prostaglandins, the inflammatory molecules which cause pain, but the great news is that turmeric and feverfew can do that job too. Fennel seeds can significantly reduce the contractions of the uterus, which is what causes the pain.

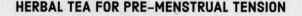

## HERBAL TEA FOR PRE-MENSTRUAL TENSION

1 tsp fresh or ½ tsp dried vervain (calming and balancing)

1 or 2 fresh rose geranium leaves (uplifting and hormone balancing)

1 slice of lemon (stimulates the liver to flush)

🌿 Drink this 2 or 3 times a day when you suffer from PMS. If you are feeling really upset and tearful, then a teaspoon each of passiflora and rose petals can really help to relax you.

## TEA FOR CONGESTIVE PRE-MENSTRUAL PAIN

½ tsp freshly grated ginger
½ tsp dried yarrow

🌿 Add to a cup of boiling water, and steep for 15 minutes.

🌿 Drink this once a day from ovulation and then if the congestion begins, raise the frequency to twice a day until menstruation.

## TEA FOR SPASMODIC PERIOD PAIN

¼ tsp freshly grated turmeric
¼ tsp freshly grated ginger
2 leaves of feverfew
½ tsp fennel seeds (crushed if you can)
a little honey (the sugar helps the
    sufferer to cope)
a sprig of mint or ¼ tsp cinnamon
    powder can be added if the
    person feels nauseous

🌿 Add all the ingredients into a teapot with a cup of boiling water. Steep for 10 minutes, strain and drink. Drink this tea up to 4 times a day until the painful days have passed.

## CRAMPING PERIOD-PAIN RELIEVING CREAM

Essential oils are wonderful friends which relieve pain, calm our emotions and help us to feel a bit more in control of our own bodies.

15 drops of lavender
5 drops of clary sage
4 drops of marjoram
10 drops of rose geranium
60g (2oz) unscented base cream, or
    you may prefer to use oil instead
    of cream, in which case 100ml
    (3½fl oz) of almond oil would be
    appropriate.

🌿 Blend together and gently rub over the lower abdomen and lower back to relieve the cramping. This can be enhanced by holding a hot water bottle over the painful area.

# ACNE

Young men, and women prior to menstruation or around the menopause, often have a little too much testosterone. This hormone can increase the sebum production of the skin. The sebum mixes with dead skin cells and can cause a skin plug in the hair follicle on the face, chest or back. Harmless bacteria which normally live on the skin feed on the sebum, causing inflammation and sometimes an infection of the skin – hence the angry red bumpy skin, often with pus.

Treating acne requires professional support, but in all cases, making sure that the liver is functioning optimally will help to metabolize the excess hormones. Once the hormones have been broken down in the liver, they are passed to the bowel for elimination, and having a congested bowel literally clogs up the works, and the skin. A simple trick is to add either chia seeds or flaxseeds to your diet, which will swell, capture the waste products and then slip them comfortably out of the bowel. My favourite is to suggest a dessertspoon of whole or freshly ground flaxseeds in a cup of yogurt, followed by a glass of warm water or herbal tea. This can be done daily and will help to cleanse the body, allowing for a better balance of the hormones.

Honey is another safe and old-fashioned remedy. When honey and water are mixed, they produce hydrogen peroxide, which is a natural antibiotic. Honey also soothes the inflamed skin. In this case, honey can be used as a soothing, anti-inflammatory and healing mask.

Cleanse your face with your favourite cleansing product, then apply raw honey to damp skin. Leave it on your face for 20 minutes, then gently wash off with warm water.

To further reduce the oiliness, you can wipe your face with a cotton wool ball soaked in witch hazel or distilled rose water. These two products tone the skin, close the pores, disable the bacteria and reduce the oiliness.

# MENOPAUSE

Some women breeze through this phase of life, but for most, it is not really a bag of laughs! Hot sweaty nights, embarrassing red-faced hot flushes during a business meeting, an unreliable memory, sometimes feeling upset for no particular reason, stiff and achy joints – just not fun. But the good news is that in my experience, the vast majority of women can be treated very successfully using herbal medicine.

The herbs are just wonderful. Within days or sometimes weeks, the symptoms fade away, either completely disappearing, or the severity and frequency so much reduced that the impact on the woman's life is negligible. She may choose to stay on her herbal prescription for several years, from time to time reducing the dose to check if she still needs them.

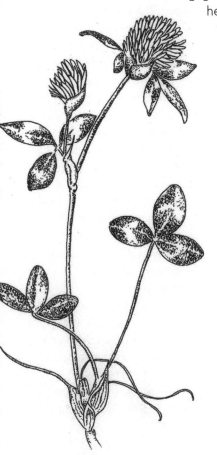

In my experience of helping women through their menopause, the herbs seem to carry them comfortably through this phase, without hot flushes, sweats or other symptoms, and then they are set down gently on the other side, to continue their lives with grace and peace.

There are herbs which a medical herbalist might choose to use, and which I cannot recommend using without professional advice (they are not dangerous, but should be used with professional knowledge), but there are others which are particularly safe and easily available, and do give great relief.

Sage, hops and red clover are all easily grown in the garden or allotment, and can be taken as a tea once or twice a day. These herbs are what we refer to as "phytoestrogenic", because they have an oestrogenic-like effect, and are appropriate for the time of life when the decline of oestrogen brings on uncomfortable symptoms.

- **Red clover** – I find this to be the gentlest (but extremely effective) herb to balance the menopausal hormones and bring the woman back to a state of harmony.

- **Sage** – Garden sage is particularly helpful for hot flushes and sweats. It is also an important herb to help support "the ageing brain" and memory.

- **Fennel** – These seeds are very easily grown in your garden or allotment, or can be purchased as tea bags from the supermarket. Fennel is rich in phytoestrogens and both experience and studies have proved this herb to be a menopausal woman's friend. It reduces hot flushes, aids sleep, and alleviates the anxiety and depression which sometimes accompany the menopause. Fennel tea can also help with vaginal dryness, although it was found to be more effective when applied as a cream.[60] Another nice bonus is that it plumps up the bust line.

- **Hops** – The green papery cones which appear at the end of summer have a delicious fruity, spicy smell. They too are rich in phytoestrogens, thus supporting declining hormone levels, but they are also specifically useful to aid sleep. Hops are also an excellent digestive aid, and when you consider that our digestive enzymatic secretions decline as we age, and that most of us eat our main meal at night, you can see how useful hops may be when taken as a tea after supper.

Menopausal women can have awful nights, where they are woken up by raging hot flushes and sweats, and then by the time they have cooled down, they are wide awake. Hops is just fabulous at reducing the severity and frequency of the flushes, because the plant contributes toward supporting oestrogen levels, whilst at the same time calming the central nervous system, allowing sleep. So even if you do have a flush, your brain is in such a peaceful state that you easily drop off to sleep again, waking in the morning refreshed and ready to take on the day. As a nice side effect, hops also plumps up the bust line.

**Motherwort** – This is a herb that I like to use with women who have a racing heart, palpitations or even anxiety associated with the menopause. It balances the hormones and the emotional system. Motherwort grows easily in the garden, and is pretty, but very fertile. I tend to cut it back before it seeds, and then there is usually a second flush of pretty pink flowers to admire. If your palpitations persist, please see your doctor.

**CAUTION:** Do not use this herb if you have a hypoactive thyroid.

*These herbs are what we refer to as "phytoestrogenic", because they have an oestrogenic-like effect, and are appropriate for the time of life when the decline of oestrogen brings on uncomfortable symptoms.*

## MENOPAUSE TEA

1 part red clover (hot flushes)
1 part sage leaves (if you suffer
    from the sweats)
1 part motherwort (if you have a
    racing heart or anxiety)
1 part dried rose petals (cooling
    and relaxing)
1 part hops cones, crushed (hot flushes
    and to help you sleep)
1 part fennel seeds (adds sweetness
    and cools hot flushes)

Make a blend of the herbs listed – all of them or some of them, according to your requirements – then take 1 teaspoon twice a day in a cup of boiling water.

## A SLEEPING INFUSION FOR MENOPAUSE

½ tsp dried valerian root, or
    Californian poppy
    (promotes sleep)
3 leaves of fresh sage (supports
    oestrogen levels)
½ tsp fennel seeds, crushed (supports
    oestrogen levels)
1 cone of hops (supports oestrogen
    levels and promotes sleep)

Add to a teapot and steep for 10 minutes, then strain and drink warm or chilled.

**A word of caution:** Phytoestrogenic herbs should not be used if you have, ever have had, or have a strong family predisposition toward hormonal-driven cancer, or any other hormonal-sensitive health conditions. Many studies show that these herbs actually protect the person from these cancers, but while the jury is still out, it is prudent to err on the side of caution.

## Cooling powders

There is always something to learn from nature. In this case, the ultimate matriarchs teach us the cooling qualities of clay. Elephants love to powder their bodies with dry clay as it keeps them cool, amongst other things. You can dust yourself off with bentonite clay to keep yourself cool and powder-dry at night.

Rose geranium has antidepressant, anxiety-reducing and calming effects, and as it smells so delightful, it makes a gorgeous dusting powder when combined with clay.[61]

~~~~~~~~~~~~~~~~~~~~~~~~~~~~~~~~

## MATRIARCH POWDER
## (IN HONOUR OF THOSE BEAUTIFUL, GENTLE AND FIERCELY PROTECTIVE ELEPHANTS)

½ cup of bentonite clay

½ cup of cornflour (cornstarch)

40 drops of rose geranium
essential oil

15 drops of lavender
essential oil

10 drops of spearmint
essential oil

🍃 Sift the cornflour and clay into a large bowl. Add the essential oils and stir with a balloon whisk, and then either a plastic or metal spoon.

🍃 Decant into a beautiful glass container, and dust yourself down with a glamourous powder puff at bedtime or any time of the day.

~~~~~~~~~~~~~~~~~~~~~~~~~~~~~~~~

## ENLARGED PROSTATE

Approximately 50 per cent of men will develop benign prostatic hypertrophy (BPH) by their mid-fifties, rising to 70 per cent in their seventies, and 90 per cent of men over 80. Like the menopause, it is not really an experience one looks forward to, but nonetheless it happens, and so we must try to mitigate the effects.

BPH is an enlargement of the prostate gland caused by a change in the sex hormone levels of the man as he ages. Responding to changing levels of oestrogen and testosterone, the gland grows, pressing on the urethra and blocking the flow of urine. The symptoms include a sense of urgency, or the inability to delay urination, incomplete emptying of the bladder which may lead to infections, frequent urination during the day and night, a weak urine stream, and sometimes incontinence.

Fortunately, there are herbs which can significantly inhibit the enlargement as well as reduce the symptoms without any ill effect on the body. Exotic herbs such as saw palmetto are excellent, and can be purchased, but this book is about herbs which you can find in your garden and the edges of fields, and they are just as good.

All three herbs would be classified by any gardener as a weed, and yet they are so helpful to humanity. One cannot help but wonder why a little weed would have the ability to change hormone levels in a human being, for surely that isn't much use to the plant itself? It must be that they are here to help us, and to me, that is an awe-inspiring concept at the very least, one which engenders huge respect and gratitude toward the plant world.

## Small-flowered willow herb (*Epilobium parviflorum*)

An assessment by the European Medicines Agency on small-flowered willowherb concluded that it offers relief of symptoms of enlarged prostate, such as frequent urination during the night and day and lack of complete bladder emptying.[62] This very common little herb barely received any attention until the Austrian herbalist Maria Treben wrote about it in the late 1970s. Since then, it has become a firm friend of men who know to use it for their prostate problems.

The famous prostate herb is saw palmetto, which comes from Florida, but it is becoming more and more expensive. The berries have a useful constituent called β-sitosterol, which reduces prostate enlargement and the associated symptoms by blocking two enzymes called 5-alpha reductase and aromatase. The former converts testosterone into the far more potent dihydrotestosterone, and aromatase converts testosterone to oestradiol, both leading to an enlarged prostate gland with the associated symptoms.

Now, rather wonderfully, our small-flowered willowherb also has within its chemical makeup β-sitosterol, which could be one of the reasons why it is so helpful for the prostate gland. So, if you want to reduce your carbon footprint and save money, you could harvest this and use it instead of saw palmetto.

## Horsetail (*Equisetum arvense*)

Traditionally horsetail herb has been prescribed for people with loss of control over their bladder, or what might be termed a "weak bladder". Whilst horsetail doesn't seem to directly affect the prostate gland, it does seem to exert a beneficial effect over some of the symptoms, namely the weak bladder and the sense of urgency. It is thought to do this by toning the tissues of the bladder wall and sphincter, quite likely through its high silica content.

Certainly, this is a herb that I have used for years when helping men with an enlarged prostate, and it has reduced the uncomfortable symptoms most admirably.

## Nettle root (*Urtica dioica radix*)

Like saw palmetto and small-flowered willowherb, nettle root is a herb which has been traditionally used to alleviate the symptoms of benign prostatic hypertrophy by slowing the growth of the prostate gland. Although not as well studied as saw palmetto, studies have confirmed that nettle root has a beneficial effect on the enlarged prostate gland.[63][64]

✿ ✿ ✿

So, here you have three herbs, all easily available, and all of which have a long tradition in supporting the health of the prostate gland, keeping older men feeling much more comfortable for years to come. If you would like to go to the effort, you can make a BPH tincture, to take every day and preserve the youthful condition of your prostate gland.

# BPH (BENIGN PROSTATIC HYPERTROPHY) TINCTURE

Collect equal quantities of nettle root, small-flowered willowherb and horsetail. Willowherb and horsetail are easy to pick, because you simply pluck off the tops. The nettle root requires a bit of digging, but you could offer an elderly friend a good service by digging up their nettles, and it is quite a satisfying job. Once dug, snip off the tops and these can be added to the compost heap if they are not in their seeding phase of life. The roots are then washed and dried off. It would be a good idea to hammer them to open the cells of the tough yellow roots because that is where the goodness lies.

Divide your herbs into three piles, then dry them for a few days so that they lose much of their water content. When you judge that they are quite dry but not snap dry, weigh each herb separately and place in a pile so that each pile weighs the same. Now place these herbs into a large Kilner jar and just cover with brandy/vodka etc.

If you don't use alcohol, then make an apple cider vinegar extract by warming some proper apple cider vinegar (purchased from a cider farmer in Somerset), and pour this over the herbs as described above.

Leave the herbs to macerate in the alcohol or vinegar for two to three weeks, and then strain into a bottle and cork. Take a wee dram of 1 tablespoon in a small glass of water, each day on an empty stomach.

## Foods which help to suppress BPH:[65]

- Soybean

- Onions

- Red wine, black grapes

- Black and green tea

- Cranberry, strawberries

- Citrus fruits

- Tomatoes, particularly cooked tomatoes

- Broccoli

- Apples

- Pumpkin seeds

- Flaxseeds

There are many hormonal conditions which are commonly treated by medical herbalists or naturopathic practitioners which I have not mentioned in this book, because they are potentially complicated and all require a proper one-to-one consultation and individualized prescription. If you have a condition which I have not mentioned, do try professional natural medicine because it aims at rebalancing your body and bringing you back to health. Mainstream medicines often dominate the body's natural rhythms, which in the long run is not helpful. Having said that, an accurate diagnosis from your GP, gynaecologist or urologist is extremely important, because some conditions can be dangerous and do need the attention of a specialist.

# CHAPTER 8

## Samhain

As the wild winds of autumn tear at the forest trees, leaves fall in skittering, spinning discs of gold onto the deep bed of the woodland floor; the gnarly limbs of the trees are exposed now. Small creatures scamper about, making preparations for the cold, dark half of the year. And on the frosty, glittering diamond-studded nights, the owls call through the forests, foxes shriek and badgers hunker down. At night, the icy fog descends, like a swirling dark anaesthetic, sinking down onto the plants, and they bow their heads in submission to the ancient crone of the year. Their green energy retreats inward toward the sanctuary of the roots, and leaves lie brown on bare earth.

Samhain is the time of the crone, the wise woman. It is the time of year when we honour our ancestors, the elderly and all the wisdom that has been gathered over the decades of life. They are the ones who really know.

It is also an opportunity to recognize our own mortality, which is sharply brought to focus through our joints, which stiffen and ache, especially during the colder part of the year as the years roll by. Once again, we call upon the wisdom of our ancestors, who knew which herbs to use in order to preserve our joints and alleviate the pain of arthritis. Let us turn yet again to the generosity of our medical plants.

> *Green energy retreats inward toward the sanctuary of the roots, and leaves lie brown on bare earth.*

# MUSCLES AND JOINTS

*ROSEHIPS* *HORSETAIL* *NETTLES* *FEVERFEW* *WHITE WILLOW* *GINGER* *TURMERIC* *DEVIL'S CLAW* *FIGWORT* *GROUND ELDER* *DANDELION LEAF* *RUE* *LAWN DAISY*

The pain of arthritis is caused by inflammation, but it is the underlying cause of the inflammation where we should focus our attention. In the case of osteoarthritis, it is the eroding of the cartilage through wear and tear which results in bone rubbing on bone. With rheumatoid arthritis, it is the immune system attacking the joint membranes. With gout, the inflammation is caused by uric acid crystals irritating the joint membranes resulting in acute and excruciating pain, and pseudo gout is a similar condition caused by calcium crystal formation.

Do not despair – there is a lot that can be done to significantly slow down the progression, and even to backtrack a little.

## OSTEOARTHRITIS

This is the type of arthritis that we all get after a certain age! It is simply the cartilage of our joints wearing out, and tends to affect the larger joints such as the knees, hips and neck. One of the most helpful things you can do for this arthritis is to lose weight (if you need to), that way reducing the burden on the joints.

To slow the progression of osteoarthritis you need to repair the cartilage as much as is realistically possible, reduce the inflammation and clear the toxic crystals from the joints, and strengthen the muscles surrounding the joint, so that they hold the limb in its correct position. There are several home remedies which can help.

## REPAIR THE CARTILAGE

Repairing the cartilage requires collagen, which can be acquired through bone broth. There are umpteen recipes on the internet to follow, so I shall leave that for you to explore. Bone broth in your food is healthy for all your tissues. It may be useful to add fresh ginger and turmeric as they are natural anti-inflammatories. Although turmeric is well known as an anti-inflammatory kitchen spice, it is also well known that curcumin, the active constituent, is difficult to absorb, and the absorption is facilitated by adding piperidine, found in black pepper. It is a simple matter of grating fresh turmeric into your bone broth and a hefty grind of black pepper to facilitate the absorption of the curcumin.

## Gelatine

As a simpler though perhaps less tasty option, it is useful to have a teaspoonful of gelatine every day. Gelatine is collagen, and has been used for aeons to supplement our own collagen, and thereby plump out skin wrinkles, strengthen hair and brittle nails, heal the gut lining and support cartilage regeneration.

A teaspoon of gelatine each day can help to slowly rebuild your joint cartilage. Gelatine can be added to stocks and soups, but the simplest way is to dissolve a teaspoon in a cup of boiling water, and add Marmite or Bovril for a savoury drink. You can also add it to your morning cup of tea, where you can't even taste it. Do make sure that you completely dissolve it, because if you try to lick it off the spoon, you will find your lips and tongue glued together – which clearly illustrates that collagen is the glue which holds our tissues together. Indeed, the word collagen comes from the Greek word "*kolla*", which means glue.

The synthesis of collagen requires vitamin C, thus rosehips, rich in vitamin C, work very well together with gelatine. If you prefer to take a vitamin C supplement, then 1g will help to enhance the quality of your skin, hair and nails, as well as boosting your immune system and cartilage repair.

**Other daily supplements which help to preserve and even rebuild cartilage include:**

- Glucosamine sulphate 1,500mg
- MSM 1,500mg
- Chondroitin 1,000mg

# Rosehips (*Rosa canina*)

Rosehips are abundantly available to be harvested on your autumnal walks along the hedgerows and other lovely unruly places. These berries were highly sought after during the war when children were sent out to collect them so that they could be turned into a syrup rich in vitamin C. You may question how much vitamin C survived after the cooking process, but apparently the vitamin C content barely dropped following the syrup-making. It is the exposure to oxygen which reduces the vitamin C content, so once chopped, work quickly.

The immune-boosting vitamin content is a nice side effect of taking these berries, but it is their anti-inflammatory, antioxidant and pain-reducing action that we are after in the case of arthritis. In 2008 a study found that rosehips were three times more effective than paracetamol and 40 per cent more effective than glucosamine.[66]

Incredibly, rosehips have been noted to have anti-diabetic and anti-obesity effects, which is precisely what is needed if we are trying to treat a weight-bearing arthritis. The wisdom of nature continues to astound me!

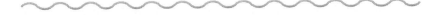

## ROSEHIP VINEGAR

I prefer to use rosehips in apple cider vinegar, partly to avoid the sugar in a syrup, and partly because apple cider vinegar is so good for you anyway.

Collect the red rosehips, rinse off, then dry. Place them in your blender. Warm (but don't overheat) the apple cider vinegar, and pour over the rosehips, then whizz until they are roughly chopped.

Pour the whole lot into a glass Kilner jar and leave to macerate for 2 weeks.

When you are ready, you must carefully strain the hips 3 times through fine muslin so that all the irritating little hairs are removed from your rosehip vinegar.

Now you can take 2 tablespoons a day in a little water as a fabulous winter tonic.

## Horsetail (*Equisetum arvense*)

Horsetail or marestail is another of those herbs that gardeners hate and herbalists love. It can never be dug up for its roots extend more than six feet under. But from deep under the Earth's surface, this ancient plant draws up the minerals, making them available for us to use.

Horsetail is about 100 million years old, one of the oldest plants on the planet. Now it is small, but back then, there were forests of *Equisetum*. Feel the plant – it is like stroking a scaly old dinosaur. What you are feeling is silica plates. It is very abundant in this mineral which is absolutely necessary for collagen formation, and helps with the strengthening of the cartilage, tendons and ligaments of our joints. Have a look at the architecture of the herb and you cannot help noticing a similarity between the plant and the bony structure of our vertebral column. The plant helps with joint problems, restoring strength and pliability to the tissues which hold our joints together.

It also has natural anti-inflammatory properties and is an excellent diuretic, which supports the action of nettles, as you will see below.

Now, if you do your research, you will discover that silica is difficult to extract, and you may well question the usefulness of horsetail if this is the case. But plants are so very clever, and nature is so very generous. The silica within the plant exists in the form of silicic acid, and this form readily diffuses into water. So now we can understand the time-honoured tradition of using this herb for bone and joint health.

Studies show that the highest silica content is to be found in September. The best way to extract this silicic acid from the herbs is by long decoction. This means that you collect your herb, bruise it in a mortar and pestle, simmer it in a covered pot of water for two hours, then switch off the heat and leave it overnight. In the morning strain the herb, throwing the exhausted plant matter onto the compost heap. The medical water can be poured into an ice-cube tray, where you can pop one out every day to drink. It is prudent not to take it every day, so do this for four weeks on, then four weeks off.

# REDUCE THE INFLAMMATION

Even though this type of arthritis is one of wear and tear, it has been discovered that almost all osteoarthritic joints have calcium crystal deposits.[67]

In the olden times, the folk were hardier than we are today, and would flick or rub their joints with bunches of nettles. This would cause blood to rush toward the affected area, washing away the spikey crystals which irritate and inflame the delicate synovial membranes. My grandmother told me that when she was young, the old people would trek off to the beekeeper to be stung. They would push their hand into the beehive, of course receiving multiple stings, and this would clear their rheumatism for several months. Today, we employ much gentler methods.

## Nettles (*Urtica dioica*)

It is theorized that nettles help to wash the calcium crystals out of the joints and the body via the kidneys, and certainly I have found that when I leave nettles out of an osteoarthritis prescription, my patient often complains.

Drinking nettle tea every day is very simple and safe. Collect young nettles in the spring, and while they are fresh, use them as such, but also dry some for the rest of the year. All you need to do is add a sprig of nettle to a cup of boiling water, allow to cool to an ambient temperature and drink. You might consider adding your ice cube of horsetail to this drink, because with the combination you will have nettle to remove the crystals and the diuretic action of both horsetail and nettle to sweep them away – and behind the scenes both are rich in silica, thus strengthening the tissues of the joint.

**CAUTION:** Avoid nettles if you have haemochromatosis, because nettles are rich in iron. On the other hand, if you have iron deficiency anaemia, drink plenty of nettle tea.

## Apple cider vinegar

For generations, people have used apple cider vinegar to dissolve and flush out calcium crystals. I cannot find any research on the efficacy of this therapy, but both my father and my partner attest to the significant improvement with their pain; one of them had even been prescribed morphine to control it. Now, two years later, you would expect the pain to be worse, but in fact, he tells me that he is experiencing less pain than ten years ago.

Apple cider vinegar is cheap and safe, and there is nothing to lose by trying this slow but seemingly sure remedy. You can expect to wait for about a year to see significant results. The dose is 2 tablespoons in a little water, sweetened with raw honey if you so wish, twice a day.

Do make sure that you use proper apple cider vinegar, because many of the brands have five per cent cider apples and the rest of the apples are discarded dessert apples. The whole process takes a long time, whereas commercial apple cider vinegar is much speeded up and the goodness is lost. I buy mine from a Somerset farmer. You can find proper apple cider vinegar on the internet.

## Feverfew (*Tanacetum parthenium*)

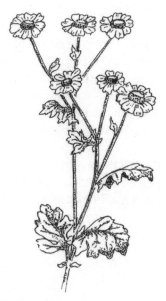

Feverfew has been called "medieval aspirin", and its species name (*T. parthenium*) comes from a legend that it saved the life of someone who had fallen off the Parthenon while it was being built.

This herb is a natural painkiller, and it achieves this by inhibiting the inflammatory molecules called prostaglandins.[68] There is a possible side effect that seems to occur in about 11 per cent of people, and that is that the herb can cause mouth ulcers, although in my practice, where I have given it as a tincture to hundreds of people, I have never heard of this side effect ever occurring. Possibly because the herb is so bitter that people immediately wash their mouth out. The old-fashioned method of taking feverfew was to add two leaves to a sandwich, and eat daily. This country remedy was used to treat arthritis and migraines, as well as period pain.

## White willow (*Salix alba*)

I once met a woman who told me a story about her willow tree and her elderly dog. She said that she had noticed every time she pruned her willow tree, her dog would dart forward and grab a stick to chew on. It took her some time to realize that after chewing on his willow stick, his mobility was much improved, and she realized that the dog was self-medicating. Since then, she always made sure that she left the willow sticks on the ground so that he could help himself as he needed. Animals are excellent at self-medicating and they know exactly how much of what to take, if only they are given the opportunity.

I digress. Let me return to us humans, who are not so good at self-medicating and tend to find most appealing that which is often bad for us!

Willow is another of nature's painkillers. It is rich in salicylates which is the stuff of aspirin, and a natural and very successful anti-inflammatory. Notice, if you will, the graceful willow. See how slender she is, and how she loves water. This gives us a clue as to the uses of willow. The bark restores flexibility to our stiff and painful limbs, especially when those limbs seize up in the cold and damp weather.

The salicylates do not easily dissolve in water, but are lipid soluble, thus an alcohol or glycerine extract would be the preferred choice of preserving this herb for the year. The salicylate levels are at their peak in March – when the sap is rising – and also September. This is the time to go hunting for willow.

## WILLOW WHISKY

Snip the slender whips from the tree (*Salix alba*), and when you take them home, sit on a chair with a wide bowl between your knees and shave off the green bark with a sharp knife. Place these shavings in a glass jar.

Now pour over the shavings a spirit alcohol such as whisky, brandy, gin or vodka, so that they are just covered. Seal the jar and leave to extract for at least 2 weeks.

After that, you can strain off the alcohol, and compost the willow. Take a wee dram of 1 teaspoon morning and evening.

**CAUTION:** Do not use willow if you are allergic to aspirin, intolerant to salicylates, or taking blood-thinning medication.

# Ginger (*Zingiber officinale*)

Ginger, as we all know, is a warming herb, rich in anti-inflammatory constituents, making it comforting for those who feel creaky during the cold and wet winter months. Ginger also has a host of other benefits, and currently there is great interest in its use for stomach or intestinal cancers, so it is no bad thing to generously include it in our diets.

# Turmeric (*Curcuma longa*)

This spice is well known by now as an anti-inflammatory herb, and indeed studies show that it is as effective as ibuprofen at reducing the pain of osteoarthritis, and without side effects. However, it is not easy to absorb. The trick is that it doesn't dissolve in water very well, and it likes to work with black pepper. Long cooking spoils its medical benefits, but gentle heating enhances absorption.

An Indian lady once told me that she gently fries turmeric powder in ghee or coconut fat with a little black pepper and includes it in her food. Another option would be to make the delicious golden milk. Traditionally, haldi doodh is made with a cup of milk and 2 teaspoons of turmeric powder, possibly sweetened with honey. Today, people enhance the flavour with cardamom and ginger, and this drink is heavenly.

## GOLDEN MILK

2 tsp turmeric powder

a good grind of black pepper

1 cup of dairy or vegetable milk
    (coconut is my favourite for
    this recipe)

1 crushed cardamom pod

a little bit of grated ginger
    (anti-inflammatory and great
    for the aches of winter)

a pinch or piece of cinnamon
    (for flavour)

honey, to taste

Warm the milk and infuse the spices for at least 10 minutes, then strain, sweeten with honey, if wished, and enjoy.

This makes a glorious bedtime drink, especially in winter.

## OSTEOARTHRITIS TEA

1 tsp gelatine

2 tbsp apple cider vinegar

1 tsp fresh horsetail (or ½ tsp
    dried horsetail)

1 sprig of fresh or dried nettle

½ tsp grated ginger

2 whole dried rosehips

2 leaves of feverfew

Add all the ingredients to a teapot and add 2 cups of boiling water. Allow to brew for 20 minutes. Drink a cup of this twice a day.

# RHEUMATOID ARTHRITIS

Rheumatoid arthritis is a tricky condition and best left for professional consultants to deal with, in conjunction with a medical herbalist and/or a nutritionist. This type of arthritis occurs when the body attacks its own tissues, leading to severe inflammation of the small joints, which can progress to permanent severe disability. The naturopathic approach is to seek out foods or intestinal parasites which may be causing inflammation of the gut lining, and gut permeability. The permeability of the gut lining allows partially or undigested food particles to enter the bloodstream, and meet the circulating immune cells. The immune system doesn't recognize these particles and does exactly what it is supposed to do: attack them. Then, the immune system becomes confused because somehow, these particles seem to be similar to our synovial membranes (the membranes which surround our joints), and so the immune system attacks its own tissues.

The conventional approach is anti-inflammatories and immune suppressors. Sometimes these are absolutely crucial. The naturopathic approach is to try to assess which foods may be causing the gut inflammation, and assiduously avoid them. We would also suggest a stool analysis to find out if there are any parasites which may be destroying the gut wall, leading to the permeability. After avoiding the foods, and restoring the correct flora and fauna to the gut, the gut lining needs to be repaired and the immune system rebalanced. All the way through, anti-inflammatory herbs would be used to minimize the damage to the synovial membranes and the joints themselves. You can see that this is a delicate operation, and really does need professional assistance.

Having said that, there are some herbs which grow wild and have proven to offer significant help – but first of all, a very simple kitchen remedy.

## Bicarbonate of soda / baking soda

In 2018, scientists from Augusta University published a study which found that by drinking 2g of bicarbonate of soda (baking soda) in

250ml (9fl oz) of water, autoimmune diseases such as rheumatoid arthritis were significantly abated.[69] [70] They discovered that the stomach was encouraged to secrete more acid, which in turn improved the digestion and breakdown of food particles.

The bicarbonate of soda (baking soda) also seems to tell the immune cells to "cool it", and not to confuse food particles with invasive bacteria. In other words, the bicarb is able to re-educate and modulate the immune system so that it does not attack its own body tissues. The scientists found that after two weeks, macrophage immune cells changed from being inflammatory to anti-inflammatory. This is a marvellous tool to use because it is safe, cheap and the science shows it is effective for a progressive disease, which is normally medicated with powerful drugs.

## Devil's claw and figwort (*Harpagophytum procumbens* and *Scrophularia nodosa*)

One of my favourite herbs for helping to reduce inflammatory joint conditions such as arthritis is devil's claw. This herb, which looks remarkably similar to a gnarly hand, grows in the extremely harsh environment of the Kalahari and Namibian deserts. It is so successful therapeutically that in France and Germany it is being considered as an alternative to non-steroidal anti-inflammatory drugs. But as is often the case, its success is its downfall, as the plant is slow-growing, in great demand and now endangered.

This is a book which focuses on the herbs and spices which you can find in your kitchen cupboard, or plants which grow in your garden or the fields, and that being the case, devil's claw could not be more exotic. However, hidden in plain sight, right here in Britain, we have a common weed, which looks nothing like *Harpagophytum* and yet has a similar concentration of harpagosides – one of the natural chemicals in devil's claw which has the anti-inflammatory effect.[71] This has led scientists to propose that figwort could be an excellent substitute for devil's claw.

Figwort (*Scrophularia nodosa*) is a diuretic and has a detoxifying action on the body, making it even more appropriate for treating arthritis naturally. What is particularly nice about using *Scrophularia* over *Harpagophytum* is that with devil's claw you have to harvest the tuber, which is extremely stressful for the environment, whereas with figwort you are harvesting the leaves of a common weed, thereby having very little environmental impact.

I do recommend you consult a medical herbalist before using this, as figwort can also stimulate the heart, so caution is needed. Having said that, scientists suggest that *Scrophularia* is well tolerated, and as a nice side effect is particularly useful for psoriatic arthritis – a condition which can be very difficult to treat.

Things can change slowly in the world of herbs. Edward the Confessor (1042–1066) introduced a ritual for a disease known as scrofula, or king's evil. The tuberculosis bacteria can cause gross swellings of the lymph nodes in the neck, groin and armpits, which may burst, releasing pus and other fluids. It was believed that the king held a divine authority to heal, and thus, the touch of the king gave an instantaneous and painless cure to this condition. In the event of the king not being available, a certain herb was used, and thus figwort acquired its botanical name, *Scrophularia*.

## Horsetail and rosehips

Horsetail has shown to have remarkable anti-inflammatory properties for rheumatoid arthritis, because it cools down the immune inflammatory process.[72] [73] [74] Rosehips, too, have been shown to reduce the inflammation of this form of arthritis, and a study showed that the rosehips reduced pain better than placebo. An analysis of several studies showed that it is the rosehip shells and seeds which were far more effective than only the rosehip shells.[75]

## GOUT

Gout was called the disease of kings and bishops, because historically it was associated with rich foods and port; however, there may also be a hereditary susceptibility. It is well known by all gout sufferers that they should radically reduce their meat and alcohol consumption, and increase their vegetable intake, but what may be less considered are the kidneys, which filter the uric acid from our blood. Gout and kidney disease are often related. There are some herbs which are wonderful diuretics, and help to wash the uric acid crystals from our body. Some of these herbs are weeds, so you can clear your weeds and your gout at the same time.

## Ground elder (*Aegopodium podograria*)

Ground elder was known as gout weed. "*Podos*" is the Greek word for foot, and you can see from the common and Latin names of this herb there is a nice association between feet, gout and this herb.

It was cultivated by the medieval monks in their physick gardens, where it became known as bishop's weed. Generally, only those who could afford plenty of meat and wine were prone to suffering from gout, and so we must assume that between the holy fasts, and wearing out their knees on cold stone church floors, the bishops ate and drank well enough to accumulate excess uric acid crystals in their joints, precipitating the necessity to call upon the aid of this humble weed. Henceforth, and even up until 1963, being the last record that I can find of this particular gout remedy, goutwort has also been used as a remedy for rheumatic joints, sciatica and haemorrhoids; a study in 2012 noted that the essential oil from the flowers had a diuretic effect which instigated the excretion of uric acid crystals.[76]

The fresh young leaves have a palatable lemony taste, not unlike coriander. Nettles taste like a richer, albeit furrier version of spinach. Since both herbs are excellent for gout, it makes sense to eat them regularly as a vegetable dish if you suffer from the condition. The Italians are familiar with cultivating nettles, and the trick for both herbs is to regularly harvest the leaves, so that the shoots remain young and tender.

## Nettles (*Urtica dioica*)

Nettles have been used for centuries to alleviate the agony of gout. Medical herbalists believe that the leaves pick up the uric acid crystals and flush them through the kidneys and out of the body. I cannot find any studies to justify this statement, but I can tell you that after years of prescribing nettles for gout, the empirical evidence suggests that it is successful and certainly worth trying.

As you can see from other chapters in this book, this herb is green gold. It is free and easily incorporated into our diets, and it is so safe! The leaves are excellent in the springtime as a detoxifying flush. Make sure that you pick them before they flower. They can be used for ravioli, soups, casseroles, omelettes, feta and nettle muffins – just use your imagination.

Collect and dry enough nettles in the spring to keep you stocked up for the winter months. During the summer, you can cultivate a "cut and come again" patch of nettles to use daily. Your dose is 1 teaspoon of fresh or dried nettles per cup of boiling water a day, or four times a day if you are under attack from gout.

## Dandelion leaf (*Taraxacum officinale*)

Dandelion leaf is a natural diuretic, helping to wash toxins and uric acid crystals out of the body. It is also a liver tonic, helping to cleanse the body by supporting the liver's natural detoxifying actions. I cannot envisage many people digging up their dandelion roots, cleaning them off, then making a meal of those roots! It is a faff. But the leaves are easy. Pick the young ones, and follow the French by adding them to your salads in the springtime.

## Celery juice

Whilst traditionally, medical herbalists use celery-seed tea to treat gout, there is research showing that the whole plant – that is the stalks and leaves – significantly reduces uric acid in the blood, which means that for home use, celery juice will do nicely. If you are suffering from a gout attack, a very simple option would be to juice an entire celery plant, and drink it in the morning before food. If you don't have a juice extractor, then chop up the celery and place in your liquidizer. Then add as little water as would be necessary to be able to blend the stalks to a mush. Pour through a sieve into a jug and drink this through the day.

## Tart cherry juice

Since the 1950s, cherry juice has been used by gout sufferers to alleviate their attacks. Studies show that by taking 30ml (1fl oz) a day, which is equivalent to 1 tablespoon twice a day of tart cherry juice concentrate, there is a 250 per cent increase in the urine excretion of urates, which translates into significantly fewer or no further attacks of gout.[77] It is important to use the tart cherry juice and not sweetened cherry juice, which has some effect but not nearly as much.

## Blackberry juice

The ancient Greeks, and more latterly, American folk medicine, used blackberries for the treatment of gout. In fact, in America, they have been called gout berries. These amazing berries are highly antioxidant, anti-inflammatory and help to remove uric acid from the bloodstream. Since blackberries are freely abundant in the hedgerows, I urge you to collect bags of these superfoods and freeze them. Each day, you can take out a handful and throw them into your smoothie or juicer to help ward off gout attacks.

## PSEUDO-GOUT

Also known as chondrocalcinosis or calcium pyrophosphate deposition (CPPD), this condition mimics gout and is incredibly painful. It is caused by the abnormal accumulation of calcium pyrophosphate dihydrate crystals in the cartilage or the joint fluid. These needle-like crystals cause inflammation and pain which is similar to gout. The underlying cause is unknown, but it is sometimes related to ageing, although high iron levels in the blood or low magnesium levels are also associated.

## Anthocyanins

Dark fruit berries such as blackberries, rosehips and cherries are very rich in a class of compound called anthocyanins, which belong to a parent class called flavonoids. These natural chemicals give the berries their dark colour, and they have many health benefits, in particular powerful antioxidant and anti-inflammatory actions, which is exactly what one needs if you have arthritic pain. Since rosehips and blackberries are abundant and freely available, it makes sense to collect as many of these berries as you can in the late summer to help with joint problems over the next year. As you have seen previously (under osteoarthritis), rosehips have a particularly positive action on inflammation of the synovial membrane.

## Apple cider vinegar

Apple cider vinegar is a well-known folk remedy for all types of arthritis, and it can be very effective for chondrocalcinosis, possibly because the natural malic and acetic acids dissolve the calcium needle-like crystals, thus significantly reducing the cause of the irritation. I have found that apple cider vinegar works slowly, but after about a year, there is a significant improvement. A year may seem like a long time, but this is an ongoing condition, so it is worth starting as soon as possible and making it part of your daily regime. I know someone who was using a walking stick and morphine for his excruciating pain, and now he has a mild twinge in his knee on a country walk, which two years ago was completely impossible.

It is very important to buy the correct type of apple cider vinegar. Check the labels, because unless it specifically states that the vinegar is made from 100 per cent cider apples, it is almost certainly made from dessert apples with a small percentage of cider apples.

I buy my apple cider vinegar from a farm in Somerset, where they grow cider apples, and the fermentation process takes three years. After a slow fermentation process, you have a living product.

## BLACKBERRY APPLE CIDER VINEGAR

🌿 Purchase 5 litres of apple cider vinegar from a cider farmer.

🌿 Collect a basketful of blackberries. Most of these will need to be frozen, and I simply pop them in a plastic tub, straight into the freezer.

🌿 Now take 2 handfuls of fresh berries, squash them up, then put them in a wide-neck glass jar. Just cover the berries with apple cider vinegar and steep for 2 weeks.

🌿 Strain it, then bottle the vinegar and keep it in the refrigerator – now that you have diluted the vinegar, you don't want it to turn horrid.

🌿 The dose is 2 tablespoons of this vinegar twice a day. If the taste is too sharp, add some raw honey.

## GOUT-RELIEF TEA

**1 tsp fresh nettle leaf**
**1 tsp fresh ground elder leaf**
**1 tsp fresh dandelion leaf (or 2 tsp of a mixture of the dried leaves)**

🌿 Add to 1 cup of boiling water, and allow to cool. Then strain and pour this infusion into your blender with a whole head of celery and whizz.

🌿 Strain the whole lot, then add 1 tablespoon of tart cherry juice concentrate, or your own homemade blackberry juice.

🌿 Drink a large glass of this twice daily on an empty stomach.

# LIGAMENT DAMAGE

When tendons or ligaments tear, they take months to heal, and can be very painful and disabling. The slowness to heal is in part due to the fact that they are without capillaries to deliver the healing nutrients, and this is where a good rub every day really helps matters. But before that, we turn to our herbs for help. There is a small garden herb which is not very well known, but was once a favourite of the convent gardens.

## Rue (*Ruta graveolens*)

Rue is known as the herb of grace, and historically was used to strengthen eyesight, or to relieve eye strain. It is a particularly powerful herb, and I kept it in my garden for years before I used it. I still do not dare use it internally, but externally, as an ointment, it is quite safe, and very effective for ligament strains.

The medical actions of rue's round blue-green leaves are many, but for our interests, they are particularly useful for strained ligaments and tendons, muscular spasm and inflammation such as a sprained ankle, twisted knee and repetitive strain injury. Homeopaths may use it for sprains and strains which are relieved by resting, the application of warmth and massage. From this, we can see that an ointment of rue could offer great relief for those in pain.

The books say that rue has an awful odour, but I really don't agree. It has a lovely green odour when rubbed, but when bruised, releases an extraordinary, deliciously fruity fragrance. I like to add essential oil of frankincense (*Boswellia serrata*), which has a peaceful, resinous fragrance, is calming, anti-inflammatory and pain-relieving.

## RUE AND FRANKINCENSE OINTMENT

Collect 2 tablespoons of rue leaves, and bruise in a mortar and pestle.

Warm some olive or almond oil in a bain-marie. If you don't have one, simply place a frying pan of water on the stove, and add boiling water. Turn to a very low heat. Now put your oil in a small saucepan, and place this in the water bath. Warm the oil and then add the crushed herb, allowing the properties of the herb material to seep into the oil for at least an hour.

Strain and discard the herb matter. Put the saucepan of oil back into the water bath and add 2 teaspoons of beeswax. Allow to melt.

Now, take a small glass pot or jar and add 20 drops of frankincense essential oil, and 20 drops of Scots pine essential oil.

Have the jar lid to hand. Carefully pour the melted ointment into the glass pot and quickly but loosely twist the lid so that you capture all the essential oils.

Allow to cool in the refrigerator; label and keep for emergencies.

This ointment can be used for strains and sprains, painful Achilles tendons, or anything related to painful ligaments and tendons, particularly where there is muscle spasm involved.

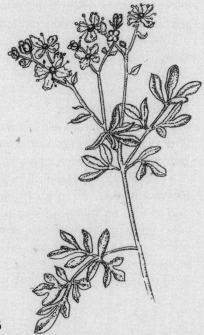

# BRUISES

Finally, the most common injury of all – bruises. We could turn to the famous, expensive and over-exploited arnica, but why would we do that when we have poor man's arnica, aka bruisewort, or lawn daisies, growing in almost every garden in the country?

## Lawn daisy (*Bellis perennis*)

This very common and delightful little flower contains saponins, which are natural blood thinners. As such, the herb helps to break down the blood which has clotted and congealed under the skin and that way shifts the bruise. *Bellis* was traditionally drunk as a tea during childbirth to reduce the pain and bruising, and is still known as bairnwort. Homeopaths use *Bellis* for deep bruises and injuries, and indeed, I love to use this herb to help people recover from surgical wounds, or those very deep bruises which take 10 days to come out and weeks to clear.

If you are bruised, recruit a kindly person to pick you a double handful of lawn daisies. Steep them in a teapot of boiling water until cool, and then either pour this in the bath and soak your bruised and battered body, or for a more focused treatment, wrap up a muslin pad, soak in the infusion and apply to the bruises directly.

For a sprained ankle, you can immerse your ankle in a foot bath of daisy infusion. I used this treatment on a badly twisted ankle once, and it reduced the pain and swelling by about 80 per cent.

### Daisies for new mums

For women, immediately following childbirth, an infusion of daisies and calendula flowers will offer great relief. You can prepare this before the birth by infusing a handful of daisy and calendula flowers in a cup of boiling water, then pouring the infusion onto a few thick sanitary towels. Wrap each pad individually in greaseproof paper and freeze, so that you have them to hand when you need them. After the birth, you can take one out of the freezer and gently press it onto the perineum area to relieve the swelling and bruising. Some women like to roll a towel into a small cushion, place the flower pad onto the towel and softly sit astride it.

As an aside, I have a lovely gypsy friend, who tells me that they used to make daisy ointment for their skin. I couldn't understand how the daisy helped their skin, until I learned that saponins also help to produce more collagen. Gypsies always know!

# MUSCLE ACHES AND PAINS

Muscles love warmth and magnesium. We live in a very stressful world, and stress draws on the adrenal glands, which in turn require magnesium and vitamin C. When we are stressed, we unconsciously draw up our shoulder muscles in a pose of self-defence. This can become habitual, and the cause of shoulder aches and headaches. Magnesium baths with warming essential oils relax the tight muscle fibres, relax our minds and ease spasmodic pain.

## MUSCLE EPSOM BATH SOAK

2 handfuls of Epsom salts
20 drops of lavender essential oil
20 drops of Scots pine essential oil
10 drops of marjoram or clary sage
    essential oil
8 drops of black pepper essential oil

Put the Epsom salts into a large bowl and add the essential oils. Mix well. Now run your bath, and only when you are in it do you toss all the salts into your bath. Lie back and relax for 20 minutes, remembering to drink cold water as you will probably be perspiring.

If you don't have a bath then you can make yourself a magnesium oil to apply after a warm shower (see page 227).

## Muscle massage

Castor oil is luscious, thick and warming, and wonderful as a massage oil for sore muscles. Because it is very thick, and has the consistency of honey, I like to combine it with olive oil, which has also been used traditionally for inflamed and sore muscles and joints. You can use these oils without essential oil, but these powerful little drops add an extra therapeutic dimension, as well as having a drifty relaxing effect on the mind.

I like to combine it with a few drops of lavender, pine and fir – you don't need much because it is very viscous. I would recommend having the massage, and then lying on your bed with a hot water bottle, wrapped in a large clean towel like a cocoon, for at least half an hour before showering the honey-like stickiness off.

## Self-massage

Well, here's the thing: home massage is something that couples can do for each other at home, but a large percentage of the population live alone – which means that their only hope of a massage is from a friend or to pay for one. Sometimes, you need a massage right now, and a foot massage is very easy and extremely comforting.

Our feet bear the weight of our lives, and as all reflexologists know, our feet hold the map of our entire body. If you live on your own, or even if you don't, it is delicious to give yourself a nurturing foot massage at the end of a long day. This is best done at bedtime so that you can relax and enjoy the benefits.

Essential oils such as Roman chamomile and lavender, or even vetiver, are calming and nourishing both to the sole and the soul.

I do encourage you not to shy away from these healing herbs for their effects are powerful, and over a few weeks, you should really notice the difference. Of course, it requires some effort to collect the herbs, but then, walking and bending is just what is needed, and next year, you can feel triumphant as you walk and bend to harvest your herbs with much greater ease.

## MAGNESIUM OIL

2 handfuls of Epsom salts
10 drops of lavender essential oil
10 drops of Scots pine essential oil
10 drops of Siberian fir or
    black spruce essential oil
10 drops of marjoram essential oil
4 drops of black pepper essential oil

Place the Epsom salts in a small saucepan, then add 200ml (7fl oz) of water. Gently heat and stir until the salts have dissolved. Allow to cool. If crystals start to form, you will need to reheat and add a little more water. Once cooled, add the essential oils.

## CASTOR AND OLIVE MUSCLE MASSAGE OIL

2 tbsp extra virgin olive oil
2 tbsp cold-pressed castor oil
4 drops of lavender essential oil
2 drops of black spruce or
    Siberian fir essential oil

4 drops of Scots pine essential oil
2 drops of marjoram essential oil
1 drop of black pepper essential oil

## CASTOR-OIL FOOT MASSAGE

Pour 1 tablespoon of castor oil into a small cup beside your bed. Add 2 drops of lavender and 2 drops of Roman chamomile.

Then massage each foot deeply. When you finish with one foot, pull a sock over it and start on the next.

Leave your socks on while you read something kind, meditate or whatever you do to wind down.

After, you can peel off the socks, but it is quite likely that you will awaken in the morning after a deep sleep, with socks on and lovely soft feet.

# NURTURING OUR EMOTIONAL STATE

### ST JOHN'S WORT ● LEMON BALM ● ROSE ● VERVAIN
### CALIFORNIAN POPPY ● LINDEN BLOSSOM ● LAVENDER
### VALERIAN ● HOPS

According to the NHS, antidepressants were the largest area of increased prescriptions in the year 2016, with a doubling of the prescriptions over a decade.[78]

This trend continued in 2019, with the *BMJ* stating that 70 million prescriptions for antidepressants were written for England in 2018, compared with 36 million in 2008.[79]

I see this trend in my practice too. While it is natural that occasionally we should experience stress or anxiety, in time we typically recover from it and continue our daily lives, living with a sense of calmness, fortitude, and hopefully joy. But these days, I see that so many people are not generally feeling happy or relaxed, or in tune with the natural cycles of life. It seems with many, there is a permanent sense of underlying anxiety. Whilst I can't help feeling that the media seems to actively promote this concept of impending doom, I often also wonder if it is because much of our society is so detached from the natural cycles of the Earth.

I think we are all relieved to note that there is a growing trend back toward the Earth, in the form of a mass exodus out of London during the coronavirus lockdown of 2020, and a massive uptake of allotments, forest bathing, forest schools and using plants as medicines. This sense of relief is interesting to me, because it suggests that we all unconsciously know that we belong to the Earth, and it is Nature who nurtures us.

We evolved with plants, and the plants are so clever at bringing us back to balance without causing addiction or doping us down. They balance our moods, our hormones, our immune system. With regard to our moods, they calm us down, so that we come back to our normal equilibrium again. Or if you have forgotten how it feels to be calm, then the herbs remind your brain that this sensation of peacefulness is how you are supposed to feel. They almost seem to reinstate our natural inner template of mental homeostasis upon which we can begin to rebuild our lives again.

As modern humans, we often strive to achieve a state of deadly calm. Life is a dynamic tension between a state of stability and creative change, and it seems that it is the change which appears to overwhelm so many. Possibly there is far too much change. Consider the speed of tech change – we can barely keep up. Perhaps we have an unrealistic expectation of stability and security, which is very nice for a while, but doesn't galvanize us into expanding ourselves into all that we can be. The trick is to find the balance, so that we can embrace and even welcome change, from a place of inner peace. Watching nature shows us that change is ever present, and it is how life is. Our resilience comes from the inner knowing that we can adapt to change and possibly even flourish when these different life experiences and opportunities are presented to us.

Herbs cannot take away emotional pain, or fear, but they can pacify an over-worried brain, or lift the spirits of a depressed mind while the owner of that mind comes to terms with, and consciously works toward, a new way of being. Plants cannot fix mental problems but they are powerful allies. In their power, they are also gentle, for they do not dominate the brain, do not dope us down. They restore balance to our neurotransmitters so that we come back to a sense of equanimity, allowing us to get on with our lives with a sense of peace and purpose.

There are so many herbs which grow in the garden, or are easily available to immediately calm the senses.

**Garden herbs which calm the nerves:** Roman chamomile, rose, lemon balm, St John's wort, lavender, valerian, hops, Californian poppy, vervain, linden blossom

**Garden herbs which uplift the spirits:** Lemon balm, rose, St John's wort, vervain, linden blossom

You will notice that there is a crossover with the calming herbs and the uplifting herbs. You may wonder how it is that a herb can bring down over-excitement, and lift under-excitement, and yet, we medical herbalists say that herbs have an amphoteric effect. They lift you up when you are low, or calm you down when you are overstimulated.

In my experience I have often found that people are not necessarily depressed but more often in despair. They may feel overwhelmed about a situation, or indeed life itself, and they can't see a way out. The anxiety which cannot find its way out turns inward to despair. After a gentle and lengthy discussion with me, or a friend, parent or professional therapist, when that person can see their way forward, their despair evaporates and a determination sets in. However, sometimes this takes time, and it is during this time that the calming or uplifting herbs can provide sanctuary for an unhappy mind while it explores its options in peace. Sometimes the person is so exhausted by their ordeal that a holistic herbal prescription is required. Anxiety can affect the skin and hair, the adrenals, the digestive system and result in chronic fatigue. Herbs help to repair the damage so that the person has the strength to make the necessary changes in their life.

*  *  *

There is far more to a medical plant than simply its chemical constituents. Why, I wonder, would a plant hold anti-anxiety chemicals within its physical body? Do plants benefit from these chemicals, or are they there simply as a gift to humans and animals? Metaphysics suggests that everything is a spark of consciousness, held in a physical vehicle. I certainly feel that is true about plants, for they seem to have conscious wisdom. Often when I am prescribing, a certain herb insists on being noticed in my mind's eye. I have learned to always include that herb, and the person always experiences a wonderful recovery. Of course the cynics will say that it is simply my unconscious mind at work. Perhaps they are correct. Perhaps not.

Most people have the idea that herbs work slowly, but in the case of anxiety and sleep they work within 20–40 minutes, and can be extremely effective.

If you have severe depression or anxiety, then it is important to see your doctor, who should arrange the correct help.

## ANXIETY AND DEPRESSION

I have often found that people who feel depressed are in a state of extreme worry. It is as if they are in a dark labyrinth of life, and they cannot see the way out. Quite often, when the person has been given the chance to talk their problems through, they are able to see the light in the dark. Even if that light is far away, they now have a goal, and in that case, some herbs to help them stay calm and strong is all they need to get them through the old door into a new way of being.

Another cause of depression can be hormonal imbalance, which is something that a medical herbalist, nutritionist or naturopath should deal with, as it requires professional consideration.

Yet another is digestive congestion. This can sound like a weird cause of depression, but you can probably imagine that someone with constipation will have lots of old food literally festering away in their gut. The toxins leach out of the bowel, and back into the bloodstream, crossing the blood-brain barrier and affecting the mood. They are also passed via the liver again, which by now is overwhelmed with toxins, possibly fat and bile sludge, and unable to eliminate them. It is not too difficult to imagine that the owner of that body will feel sluggish, have low moods and headaches and feel irritable. Once the bowel is moving again, and the liver is cleansed, you have a brighter person with their sparkle back. Just like a clogged-up river system, which has been unblocked once again.

## St John's wort (*Hypericum perfoliatum*)

My herbal medicine teacher was a wise old man, and he taught us that St John's wort is not just an antidepressant, but should be used for those who have been so stressed for so long that it is as if their nerves have been stripped bare. St John's wort is what we call a nervous tropho-restorative. It heals and restores nervous tissue and function, not only mentally but physically too.

St John's wort should be picked on or around St John's Day, which is 24 June, one of the three days of the Summer Solstice. The flower is a close representation of our sun, radiating warmth and light to our Earth, just as the plant brings warmth and light to us during our times of darkness. Around this date every year, my partner Adrian and I make the pilgrimage high up into the hills around my house to collect St John's wort, growing in amongst dog roses, wild mountain thyme and tall spires of yellow agrimony. The hills are alive with birds swirling above, and flittering butterflies who will not stop long enough for us to photograph, and dogs barking joyfully somewhere far away. It is indeed one of our most joyful jobs of the year.

St John's wort can be used as a tea or turned into a tincture or oxymel. By balancing our serotonin levels, this herb both calms our chattering anxiety and lifts gloomy spirits. It also dampens down the pain pathways in the brain, helping to relieve nerve pain, and is a powerful antiviral herb, making it perfect for neuralgia caused by shingles.

In Germany, this herb is used mainly as a liver tonic, and this is relevant to our emotional state, because depression can also be caused by a congested liver which is unable to adequately process the hormones and toxins out of the body. Thus, the hormones and toxins back up, clouding our brain and sometimes resulting in an inner rage, which we dare not express, and again, this turns inward into despair and depression.

St John's wort is a somewhat controversial herb which gets a lot of bad press. A plant contains within its chemical makeup hundreds and possibly even thousands of constituents, which work together like an orchestra. When a nutraceutical company decides that one of those hundreds of constituents is the chemical which has the antidepressant effect, and then produces a product which massively increases that single constituent but contains almost none of the other balancing constituents of the whole plant – you have a man-made medicine presenting itself as a herbal product. The balance is completely thrown out and there can be dangerous consequences. A medical herbalist will always use "whole plant extract". That means that nothing is added or removed; the plant is extracted as it is found in nature, and the result is a gentle, balanced healing. A herbalist's adage says that "The plant is more than the sum of its parts", and it is true. We also say that the plant is made up of lots of constituents and a bit of magic, because plant healing has intelligence. Somehow, the plant knows how to heal us, and it is not just a certain chemical having a certain effect on a particular organ. There is more to herbal healing than just chemistry, but we don't know what it is. Suffice to say that nature is amazing.

I urge you to keep it gentle when it comes to herbs. The plants are powerful in their gentleness and the healing is profound.

**CAUTION:** St John's wort should not be used if you are taking antidepressant or sedative medication, or contraceptives. I would advise avoiding St John's wort if you are taking any medication, unless prescribed by a medical herbalist, or in agreement with your doctor.

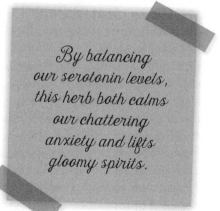

By balancing our serotonin levels, this herb both calms our chattering anxiety and lifts gloomy spirits.

## Lemon balm (*Melissa officinalis*)

Melissa is easily grown in any garden, and quickly becomes a fair-sized bush, imparting its gentle lemony fragrance to a summer's garden. The herb is useful for those who have a slightly overactive thyroid, which can give the symptoms of anxiety and palpitations, but it is also useful for everyday anxiety. Remember that with anxiety, there will be an overstimulated sympathetic nervous system, and elevated cortisol levels, which can have a depressing impact on our immune system, making us vulnerable to viral infection. Nature is very clever, and very generous. Lemon balm happens to be a very effective relaxing herb, whilst at the same time has excellent antiviral properties. As a tea, this plant is particularly refreshing and pleasant; it not only calms the nerves but also uplifts the spirits, making it perfect for anxiety as well as mild depression.

I once had a visitor who arrived at my home puce with agitation. In those days I didn't keep any herbs at home, and so all I could offer was a cup of lemon balm tea, and within half an hour, he was asleep in the chair.

Lemon balm does not dry well, as it loses all its fragrance. It is best taken as a fresh tea.

**CAUTION:** Avoid lemon balm if you have a hypoactive thyroid.

## Rose (*Rosa damascena*)

The volatile oils of roses are the chemicals giving the rosy fragrance and have been shown to reduce high levels of adrenaline and cortisol, but this is a herb particularly suited for anxiety of the heart. Rose has always been the flower of the heart. In Iran, rose water is scattered at weddings as a symbol of love and purity, and is also used to aid meditation and prayer at mourning ceremonies to calm and relax people.

It is interesting that grief often goes to our lungs too. Traditional Chinese medicine says it is related to the taking in and letting go of air and our emotions. Of course, we feel that terrible aching constriction and difficulty breathing when we are in deep grief. Now research has shown us that rose does indeed have a relaxing effect on the mind, and also on the muscles of the bronchi. What is important is that it is the fat-soluble volatile oils which have these effects, which means that the essence of rose is best captured through inhalation in a herbal infusion. This is very effective as the fragrance rises up through the nose, straight into the emotional centre of the brain called the limbic system, where emotions can be processed and healing can begin.

What a lovely thing it is, if feeling upset, to sit in a beautiful garden and drink a herbal tea of rose petals and lemon balm. Use a sprig of lemon balm and the petals of a fragrant (but unsprayed) rose.

## ROSE PETAL GLYCERINE
**One of the ways I love to preserve rose petals for medicine is to push the petals into a jar of vegetable glycerine.**

After 3 days, I strain and remove the old petals, and then add fresh petals. I do this over and over again, until by the end of summer, I have a bottle of rich rosy glycerine, which is smooth, sweet and comforting for those of my patients in emotional distress.

A teaspoon of this glycerine can be mixed with some warm water and sipped as required.

## Vervain (*Verbena officinalis*)
Vervain is a small and very inconspicuous little plant, and yet, it has been one of the most sacred herbs in the ancient world. It is also a herb of mystery because no one seems to know exactly why it was so sacred. Known to the Romans as *herba sacra*, the herb of grace or the divine weed, they made little brooms of vervain and swept the alter of Jupiter, the god of sky, thunder and protection.

Pliny tells us that if a dining hall were sprinkled with vervain-steeped water, then all around the "table would be very pleasant and make merry very jocundly".

The ancients dedicated her to Venus, and brides would pluck a sprig on the morning of their wedding day to guarantee a happy marriage.

Looking at the history of this lovely little herb, it seems to be much associated with joy and love, and it would seem that however we choose to imbibe it, that happiness will enter our lives. The ancient Druids harvest this herb with great ceremony, always leaving a libation of honeycombs in gratitude and payment for the precious gift of the herb. Whenever I harvest vervain, I always leave some honey in a jar for the ants, who take it underground and give it to the Earth.

## VERVAIN VINEGAR

Cut the pale blue flower stalks at the height of summer, snip into tiny pieces, and place in a glass jar. Gently warm some apple cider vinegar, then pour it over the herb, making sure that all of the herb is covered.

Gently shake the jar daily, and after 2 weeks you can strain and retain the herbal vinegar. Of this vinegar, take 1 tablespoon daily in a cup of warm water, and add a little honey to sweeten if you desire.

## A BEAUTIFUL INFUSION
## TO SOOTHE DISTRESS AND SADNESS

a sprig of lemon balm
a sprig of vervain
fresh rose petals (preferably from
  the Damascus rose)
a little honey (preferably heather
  honey, for heather is associated
  with the bees bringing the
  sweetness of life into the home)

Place the herbs in a teapot and pour boiling water over them, then quickly close the lid. After a few minutes, you can pour and enjoy, making sure to inhale the beautiful aromas too, because these are immediately beneficial to the mind.

## Californian poppy (*Eschscholzia californica*)

Cali poppy is a plant very well suited to pot growing and offers the most gorgeous silky orange-yellow flowers to brighten us up. It works by soothing the nerve impulses to the brain and in doing so, reduces pain, spasms, anxiety and difficulty sleeping. It is so safe that I have even used it to help babies sleep. After valerian, this is my number one go-to herb for sleep and anxiety. You can simply add 1 teaspoon of chopped Californian poppy flowers to a cup of boiling water, with a little honey, and sip. For babies, use ⅕ teaspoon of flowers to a cup of water, and add 1 or 2 tablespoons of this infusion to their bottle.

## The chamomiles

There are two main types of chamomile. The German chamomile (*Matricaria recutita*) is the one found in tea bags, and the Roman chamomile (*Anthemis nobilis*) is less commonly available in the shops but easy to grow. Although both are calming, I differentiate with Roman chamomile as my preferred relaxing herb, and German chamomile as my preferred anti-inflammatory and anti-spasmodic herb for the gut.

One of the main constituents in the volatile oil of Roman chamomile is angelic acid (imagine that! From the angels themselves), which is a sedative, and accounts for the peaceful effect that this flower has on our nervous system. Not much is needed: only a flower head or two in a cup of boiling water (always cover the cup with a lid to keep the angelic volatile oils from escaping). This tea is so gentle that it can easily be used to calm a fractious baby.

When children get upset, I often notice that it goes to their tummy. They may not even realize that they are upset, but they will say that they have a sore tummy. In this case the German chamomile can soothe the spasms of the intestinal tract.

If you feel the need to further soothe the child, add a fresh or dried flower head of Roman chamomile to a cup of chamomile tea and a little honey. This should calm the little one nicely. If you don't have Roman chamomile but have Californian poppy in your garden, try one of those gloriously golden flowerheads in the tea.

## Linden blossom (*Tilia cordata*)

If you don't have a garden, you almost certainly have a park near to you, and within that park you will probably find towering linden trees. In summer, you will find these dripping in the honeydew which is produced by millions of aphids feeding on the sap. The aphids are, in turn, profitably farmed by ants for their sweet honeydew. Bees love the flowers too, and simply lying under one of these giants on a warm summer's day, with the soporific hum of the bees collecting nectar, is a pleasantly dizzying experience. Take some of the bliss home with you by collecting a small basket of the gloriously fragrant flowers and either make a gentle tea from them or bathe in them. To do this, you must make a strong tea of the flowers in a large teapot. Once extracted for 20 minutes, add to your bath for a fragrant and peaceful experience. If you don't have a bath, perhaps enjoy a foot bath.

## Lavender (*Lavandula angustifolia*)

Our grandmothers knew to reach for the lavender when life got a bit too much, but we seem to have nearly forgotten that; yet lavender does have a significantly calming effect on our minds. Two clinical trials showed oral lavender to be equally as effective as benzodiazepines in a programme lasting seven weeks for sufferers of generalized anxiety disorder, but the dose was taken as a capsule of essential oil and most of us don't have access to those capsules.[80] [81]Taking essential oils orally is more common in Europe; however, we can dot the oil on our skin or clothing to have a very similar effect because our emotional brain, the limbic system, is positioned right above our nasal passages, and so the essential oils which we inhale diffuse directly into the emotional brain and the effect is immediate.

In another study, 200 dental patients were offered the same music and the same background décor in the waiting room, but one group was offered either orange or lavender essential oil in the room, whilst the other group had no essential oils in the room. The final analysis showed that both essential oils reduced anxiety and improved the moods of the patients when compared to the control group.[82]

Lavender can be enjoyed either as an infusion, an essential oil or as a tincture. As it is highly aromatic and this has a relaxing effect on the nervous system whilst stimulating the digestive juices, I love to use lavender with people who are so wound up that they cannot digest their food. Most people don't realize that they are in this state, but common symptoms such as excess flatulence, bloating and an irritable bowel may suggest anxiety leading to inhibited secretion of digestive acids. Check with your doctor first, however, just in case you have another underlying condition.

## Valerian (*Valeriana officinalis*)

Valerian is one of my favourite herbs, and probably the most popular herb in my dispensary. The first time I stepped into an apothecary, the room was suffused with the fragrance of valerian (as all apothecaries are), and I knew that I had found my place in the world. I have used this herb to help thousands of people who feel so uptight that they cannot think clearly, or their busy mind will not allow them to drop off to sleep. Valerian does not dope you out; instead it keeps the brain calm and clear. It quietens your brainwaves so that you can calmly get on with your strategic day, or make your presentation without feeling so tense that you can't think clearly, and soothes an overactive mind so that you tip into a deep and restful sleep.

*Valeriana officinalis* is a beautiful plant and will seed prolifically. It grows into tall spires with dainty pink-lilac flowers. The root is the medicinal part, and this is the tricky bit, because you need to dig up the plant, wash off the roots, then chop them into small pieces before drying. Then you can use the dried roots for tea. I don't grow my own valerian supplies, because it is such a popular herb in my dispensary that I would require a farm to produce all the valerian that I use each year.

For domestic use, if you can cultivate a patch, then in the autumn, you need to dig up the roots. Replant the little ones for next year. Cut off the tops, wash the mud off the roots, and dry in a cool place. Make sure you keep the root safe from your cat, who will delight in rolling joyfully in a nest of valerian root, and possibly become quite possessive of it and aggressively refuse to hand it back over to you.

My partner Adrian had the most fabulous ginger cat called Damien, who reached a venerable age of 24. Damien didn't easily share his affections, but I won him over by always bringing him presents whenever I visited, and his favourite gift was a stem of valerian with the root attached. This he loved to bat about, roll in, gnaw on, and it generally put him into a very good mood, and me into his good books.

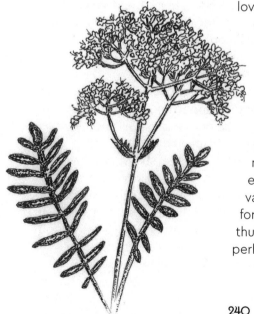

**CAUTION:** In a small but significant percentage of people, valerian agitates the person, or makes sleep even more impossible. If you have ever experienced this with valerian then this is not the herb for you, because it will ever be thus. Try another herb instead – perhaps Californian poppy or hops.

# Hops (*Humulus lupulus*)

Hops is quite easily grown in a garden over a sturdy structure, but it is as easy to spot in old hedgerows, probably as an escapee from old hop fields. It is the cones that we are after, and they are produced in the very late summer/early autumn. These soft green cones smell deliciously spicy, and yet they lull us off to sleep.

Hops pillows are famously used to induce sleep in the insomniac. I once made one, but it made my sleep worse, because the papery cones crackled all night as I moved my head. Hops pillows are better when used under a normal sleeping pillow.

Hops is one of my favourite herbs as it has several actions which are extremely helpful. It is a bitter herb – thus it stimulates the secretion of digestive acids. It is very calming to the nervous system, and it has an oestrogenic-like effect, and thus I use it for three particular conditions: for irritable bowel syndrome, when the person is so anxious that their parasympathetic nervous system (rest and digest) is dominated by the sympathetic nervous system (fight or flight) and so their ability to digest their food is much diminished; for menopausal women who can't sleep for their hot flushes; and for those who can't drop off to sleep.

## LAVENDER BEDTIME MILK

1 flower head of lavender
1 cup of milk (almond, oat or dairy)
a little honey

🌿 Warm the milk, add the flower and stir in the honey, then take this to bed.

## SLEEPY–TIME TEA

1 bag of valerian tea, or ½ tsp dried
   Californian poppies
1 hops cone

🌿 Pour a cup of boiling water over the herbs, steep and drink. This is not a delicious tea, but you will drop off into the most peaceful sleep.

# EPILOGUE

# All Time from Ecotherapy to Ecophilia

We belong to the Earth. The Earth does not belong to us. We are made of the same stuff as everything else that grows, walks, crawls, swims or flies upon this Earth.

Our bones are made from the minerals of the local soil and water. Our blood is enriched with the oxygen respirated from the trees surrounding our homes. Atoms from the stars came to Earth, once crossed great oceans, passed through the bodies of countless sea creatures, rose up to the clouds and fell back down again on their journey through your body, and once again into the Earth's body. All of nature is one, and we all need each other. When we pay attention, our souls remind us of this.

One night, when I was almost grown up, I sat with a tiny band of friends on the sandy shore of a lagoon along the Garden Route of South Africa. Our families had been on a trip to the Kruger National Park, and stopped over for a few days at Sedgefield. We were due to return home the next day, but that night, us kids had gone down to the beach, lit a fire, and were lolling around chatting and smoking cigarettes pilfered from our parents, as kids do. The night sky was like diamond-studded velvet, with warm soft sand beneath us and the rhythmic crashing waves in the near distance, the stillness of the lagoon right next to us. There were monkeys in the trees on the island just over the water, and we knew sharks patrolled the waters of that wild sea right next to us.

Suddenly and completely unexpectedly, I was struck with a heart-wrenching lovesickness. I was in love with the land, and as heartbroken as one would be when torn from their beloved. I yearned with all my heart to become one with the Earth. I wanted to be a grain of sand, the moonlight, the mist over the cliffs. To this day I feel that my soul wriggled into that sand like an invisible seed and sent roots down there forever. Now I know that my heart is in England, but my soul belongs to Africa.

Another time, walking in the Knysna forest – the last remnants of a primordial forest in the far south of Africa, where elephants still live in secret – I was searching for the elephants, which of course I didn't find. But I sat down and listened to the trees. I heard them creak and groan to me, "Help us". I was struck down by my youthful loss as to know what to do. For years, I didn't know how to fulfil my promise to help them, but now I write books and run workshops in the hope of facilitating that falling in love with nature: ecophilia.

I hope that those trees know. In theory they should, for according to quantum physics, we are all connected. The universe was once the size of a pea, and all the atoms of the entire universe were in that pea. The slow big bang occurred, and the universe continues to expand. Quantum physics shows us that if atoms were once connected, then even if separated by time and space, what happens to one atom will affect the other. This even affects scientific experiments where the observer cannot be neutral, and the atoms behave differently when observed as when not observed, because we are all connected. Thus, those big trees in the Knysna forest must know that I am helping them in my way.

A shamanic-like personage once stated that we will be lonely when the animals have gone. I was filled with a sense of dread when I heard that, because I truly believe that whilst we don't particularly wish to bump into a lion, the thought of them all gone fills us with a desperate sense of broken-heartedness.

The same for the trees. When we learnt of ash die-back, it made us sad. I thought of that great world tree Yggdrasil, the cosmic tree of the Vikings. When that dreadful serpent Nidhogg has finally chewed through the roots, Yggdrasil will fall, and that will be the time of Ragnarok – the chaotic End-Time.

I can only assume that humans want to preserve nature. We know that we have a certain feeling of wellbeing when we spend time in it. I am conscious of a deep longing within modern humans to return home, to nature. Modern living so divorces us from the Earth that many people are seeking, but cannot find that path home – yet the paths are right in front of us, in our everyday life.

New concepts of eco holidays and eco therapy such as forest bathing and wild swimming are hugely popular, and they in themselves are a powerful path back to nature. One used to be considered a bit "sandals and brown rice" if you admitted to tree hugging, but now meditating with a tree is pretty mainstream. We can listen to plants "singing" through incredible devices such as Music of the Plants, or PlantWave.

Spiritual groups such as Druidry represent one of the fastest growing non-faith spiritualities as people are attracted to the idea of nature being sacred – as it seems our ancient ancestors once were, and indigenous folk throughout the world still are.

Even in our mundane everyday life, we can use our vegetables to reconnect to nature. Just noticing what is going on in your vegetable tray can open your heart to the world of plants. Back in the 1960s Cleve Backster demonstrated that plants have intelligence and respond to events and human intention. Backster was an interrogation specialist for the CIA, and he used a polygraph (a lie-detector) to investigate whether plants could be used in crime scenes. He found that plants could "read the intentions" of humans, and when they planned to eat or harm the plant, the polygraph would flatline, as if the plant had fainted.

Now, as I look at my vegetables, I notice how they grow rootlets if left too long in the refrigerator, or how quickly asparagus grows upward toward the sun if I put it in a jar of water on the windowsill. Even fresh turmeric, all the way from India, can still sprout a green shoot if left long enough in the spice tray. They are not dead. They are still actively living beings seeking to continue expressing their life force. I once kept a leek so long that it started to produce a flower bud, and I couldn't bear to boil it alive. I planted this one in the garden so that it could complete its life cycle, and I enjoyed watering my leek.

Naturally, you cannot do that with all your vegetables because we need to eat, but we can thank our vegetables for the life force which they impart to our bodies. We can slice off the bottom of our cauliflower and put it in a vase of water on the windowsill for a day or two, with the intention that it may live its last day or two in comfort, and on some level, may know that you are grateful for its sacrifice.

Home herbal medicine is another path back to nature. Growing your own herbs, or going out into the hedgerows and forest edges to collect wild leaves and berries, bringing them home and making them into your own medicine, is a powerful way to reconnect with nature. You tune into the rhythm of the year as you watch for the leaves, flowers and berries which ripen at certain times of the year. I call it the hedgerow clock. Harvesting these herbs slows us down, we get a little nettle stung, rose-thorn scratched and maybe a bit sun-blushed, but these injuries feel good. They are a part of rewilding yourself. You fall into "flow" as you harvest, and later you experience the incredible power of nature, and her gentle non-dominance over your body as she heals you and your family. Home herbal medicine is an enchanting path back home, to Mother Nature, Gaia, our beautiful blue planet Earth.

> *Herbal medicine is an enchanting path back home, to Mother Nature, Gaia, our beautiful blue planet Earth.*

# BIBLIOGRAPHY

1 Roschek B Jr, Fink RC, McMichael MD, Li D, Alberte RS. Elderberry flavonoids bind to and prevent H1N1 infection in vitro. *Phytochemistry*. 2009 Jul; 70(10):1255–61. doi: 10.1016/j. phytochem.2009.06.003. Epub 2009 Aug 12. PMID: 19682714. 28/01/21

2 www.pharmacytimes.com/contributor/cate-sibley-pharmd/2017/10/elderberries-a-potent-cold-and-flu-remedy. Cate Sibley, PharmD. 28/01/21

3 Krawitz, Christian et al. "Inhibitory activity of a standardized elderberry liquid extract against clinically-relevant human respiratory bacterial pathogens and influenza A and B viruses." *BMC complementary and alternative medicine vol. 11 16. 25 Feb. 2011*, doi: 10.1186/1472–6882–11–16.

4 news.unair.ac.id/en/2020/03/20/studying-the-benefits-of-turmeric-and-curcuma-unair-expert-they-improve-immune-system/. 28/01/21

5 Praditya, Dimas et al. "Anti-infective Properties of the Golden Spice Curcumin." *Frontiers in microbiology vol. 10 912. 3 May. 2019*, doi: 10.3389/fmicb.2019.00912

6 Afagh Moataria, et al. "The Antiinfluenza Virus Activity of Hydroalcoholic Extract of Olive Leaves". *Iranian Journal of Pharmaceutical Sciences. Summer 2006*: 2(3): 163–168

7 Jozsef Haller, Judit Hohmann, Tamas F Freund. The effect of Echinacea preparations in three laboratory tests of anxiety. Comparison with chlordiazepoxide. *Phytotherapy Research, Wiley*, 2010, 24 (11), pp.1605. ff10.1002/ptr.3181ff. ffhal-00589442f

8 James B. Hudson, "Applications of the Phytomedicine Echinacea purpurea (Purple Coneflower) in Infectious Diseases", *BioMed Research International, vol. 2012*, Article ID 769896, 16 pages, 2012. doi.org/10.1155/2012/769896

9 Efficacy of Natural Honey Treatment in Patients with Novel Coronavirus. https://clinicaltrials. gov/ct2/show/NCT04323345. 28/01/21

10 Sangiovanni E et al, "Ellagitannins from Rubus berries for the control of gastric inflammation: in vitro and in vivo studies". *PLoS One. 2013 Aug 5*; 8(8):e71762. doi: 10.1371/journal.pone.0071762. PMID: 23940786; PMCID: PMC3733869.

11 Danaher, Robert J et al. "Antiviral effects of blackberry extract against herpes simplex virus type 1. "*Oral surgery, oral medicine, oral pathology, oral radiology, and endodontics vol. 112,3 (2011)*: e31–5. doi: 10.1016/j.tripleo.2011.04.007

12 Mazumder, Anisha & Dwivedi, Anupma & Du Plessis, Jeanetta. (2016). Sinigrin and Its Therapeutic Benefits. *Molecules. 21. 416. 10.3390/molecules21040416.*

13 Hadjivassiliou M et al. Gluten sensitivity as a neurological illness. *Journal of Neurology, Neurosurgery & Psychiatry 2002*; 72:560–563

14 Pruimboom L, de Punder K. The opioid effects of gluten exorphins: asymptomatic celiac disease. *J Health Popul Nutr. 2015*; 33:24. Published 2015 Nov 24. doi: 10.1186/s41043-015-0032-y

15 Socci, Valentina et al. "Enhancing Human Cognition with Cocoa Flavonoids." *Frontiers in nutrition vol. 4 19. 16 May. 2017*, doi: 10.3389/fnut.2017.00019

16 Nehlig A. The neuroprotective effects of cocoa flavanol and its influence on cognitive performance. *Br J Clin Pharmacol. 2013*; 75(3):716–727. doi: 10.1111/j.1365–2125.2012.04378.x

17 Lopresti AL. Salvia (Sage): A Review of its Potential Cognitive-Enhancing and Protective Effects. *Drugs R D. 2017*; 17(1):53–64. doi: 10.1007/s40268-016-0157-5

18 Luvone T et al. The spice sage and its active ingredient rosmarinic acid protect PC12 cells from amyloid-beta peptide-induced neurotoxicity. *J Pharmacol Exp Ther. 2006 Jun*; 317(3):1143–9. doi: 10.1124/jpet.105.099317. Epub 2006 Feb 22. PMID: 16495207.

19 O.V. Filiptsova, L.V. Gazzavi-Rogozina, I.A. Timoshyna, O.I. Naboka, Ye.V. Dyomina, A.V. Ochkur,

The essential oil of rosemary and its effect on the human image and numerical short-term memory, *Egyptian Journal of Basic and Applied Sciences, Volume 4, Issue 2, 2017*, Pages 107–111

20  Sayorwan, Winai et al. "Effects of inhaled rosemary oil on subjective feelings and activities of the nervous system." *Scientia pharmaceutica vol. 81,2 (2013)*: 531–42. doi: 10.3797/scipharm.1209–05

21  O.V. Filiptsova et al. The effect of the essential oils of lavender and rosemary on the human short-term memory, *Alexandria Journal of Medicine, Volume 54, Issue 1, 2018*, Pages 41–44, ISSN 2090–5068, https://doi.org/10.1016/j.ajme.2017.05.004.

22  Elena Franco-Robles et al, Effects of curcumin on brain-derived neurotrophic factor levels and oxidative damage in obesity and diabetes. *Applied Physiology, Nutrition, and Metabolism, 23 August 2013*, doi.org/10.1139/apnm-2013-0133

23  Farahanikia, Behnaz et al. "Phytochemical Investigation of Vinca minor Cultivated in Iran." *Iranian journal of pharmaceutical research: IJPR vol. 10,4 (2011)*: 777–85.

24  Patyar S, Prakash A, Modi M, Medhi B. Role of vinpocetine in cerebrovascular diseases. *Pharmacol Rep. 2011*; 63(3):618–28. doi: 10.1016/s1734–1140(11)70574–6. PMID: 21857073.

25  Zyryanova et al. White Birch Trees as Resource Species of Russia: Their Distribution, Ecophysiological Features, Multiple Utilizations *Eurasian Journal of Forest Research, 13(1), 25–40. Issue Date 2010–08*. Doc URL hdl.handle.net/2115/43853. Hokkaido University

26  Arata, Satoru et al. "Continuous intake of the Chaga mushroom (Inonotus obliquus) aqueous extract suppresses cancer progression and maintains body temperature in mice." *Heliyon vol. 2*, 5 e00111. 12 May. 2016, doi: 10.1016/j.heliyon.2016.e00111

27  www.phytoncides.org/phytoncide-phytoncides.html. As of 29/01/21.

28  Li Q et al. Effect of phytoncide from trees on human natural killer cell function. Int J Immunopathol Pharmacol. *2009 Oct-Dec*; 22(4):951–9. doi: 10.1177/039463200902200410. PMID: 20074458.

29  Lou Z et al. The effect of burdock leaf fraction on adhesion, biofilm formation, quorum sensing and virulence factors of Pseudomonas aeruginosa. *J Appl Microbiol. 2017 Mar*; 122(3):615–624. doi: 10.1111/jam.13348. Epub 2017 Jan 18. PMID: 27860087. As of 20/01/21.

30  Miazga-Karska M et al. Anti-Acne Action of Peptides Isolated from Burdock Root-Preliminary Studies and Pilot Testing. *Molecules. 2020 Apr 27*; 25(9):2027. doi: 10.3390/molecules25092027. PMID: 32349230; PMCID: PMC7248785.

31  Rani N, Vasudeva N, Sharma SK. Quality assessment and anti-obesity activity of Stellaria media (Linn.) Vill. *BMC Complement Altern Med. 2012 Sep*; 12 145. doi: 10.1186/1472–6882–12–145. PMID: 22943464; PMCID: PMC3468403. As of 29/01/21

32  Ma L et al. Anti-hepatitis B virus activity of chickweed [Stellaria media (L.) Vill.] extracts in HepG2.2.15 cells. *Molecules. 2012 Jul 18*; 17(7): 8633–46. doi: 10.3390/molecules17078633. PMID: 22810196; PMCID: PMC6268626.

33  Dr. Paschotta R. The Photonics Spotlight > 2007–02–16. *The Science of Biophotons*. Posted on 2007–02–16 (revised on 2011–05–09) www.rp-photonics.com/spotlight_2007_02_16.html. As of: 01/02/21

34  www.esalq.usp.br/lepse/imgs/conteudo_thumb/Are-humans-really-beings-of-light.pdf. As of 01/02/21

35  Dotta BT, et al. Increased photon emission from the head while imagining light in the dark is correlated with changes in electroencephalographic power: support for Bókkon's biophoton hypothesis. *Neurosci Lett. 2012 Apr 4*; 513(2):151–4. doi: 10.1016/j.neulet.2012.02.021.

36  Nelson R (200), Coherent Consciousness and Reduced Randomness: Correlations on September 11, 2001, *Journal of Scientific Exploration, Vol. 16, No. 4*, pg 549–570.

37  Orme-Johnson D W, Fergusson, L. (2018). Global impact of the Maharishi Effect from 1974 to

2017: Theory and Research. *Journal of Maharishi Vedic Research Institute, 8, 13–79*, research.miu. edu/maharishi-effect/

38   Frigolet ME, Gutiérrez-Aguilar R. The Role of the Novel Lipokine Palmitoleic Acid in Health and Disease. *Adv Nutr. 2017*; 8(1):173S-181S. Published 2017 Jan 17. doi: 10.3945/an.115.011130

39   Özcan, Tamer. (2008). Some vitamin and organic acid contents in the fruits of Prunus spinosa L. subsp. dasyphylla (Schur) Domin from Europe-in-Turkey. *IUFS Journal of Biology Research Article J Biol*. 105. 105–114.

40   Allio A et al. Bud extracts from Tilia tomentosa Moench inhibit hippocampal neuronal firing through GABAA and benzodiazepine receptors activation. *J Ethnopharmacol. 2015 Aug 22*; 172:288–96. doi: 10.1016/j.jep.2015.06.016. Epub 2015 Jul 2. PMID: 26144285.

41   Khan AU, Gilani AH. Blood pressure lowering, cardiovascular inhibitory and bronchodilatory actions of Achillea millefolium. *Phytother Res. 2011 Apr*; 25(4):577–83. doi: 10.1002/ptr.3303. Epub 2010 Sep 20. PMID: 20857434.

42   Acar-Tek N, Ağagündüz D: Olive Leaf (Olea europaea L. folium): Potential Effects on Glycemia and Lipidemia. *Ann Nutr Metab 2020*; 76:10–15. doi: 10.1159/000505508

43   Cheurfa M, Abdallah HH, Allem R, Noui A, Picot-Allain CMN, Mahomoodally F. Hypocholesterolaemic and antioxidant properties of Olea europaea L. leaves from Chlef province, Algeria using in vitro, in vivo and in silico approaches. *Food Chem Toxicol. 2019 Jan*; 123:98–105. doi: 10.1016/j.fct.2018.10.002. Epub 2018 Oct 4. PMID: 30292622.

44   Najafian, Younes et al. "Plantago major in Traditional Persian Medicine and modern phytotherapy: a narrative review." *Electronic physician vol. 10,2 6390–6399*. 25 Feb. 2018, doi: 10.19082/6390

45   Roschek B Jr, Fink RC, McMichael M, Alberte RS. Nettle extract (Urtica dioica) affects key receptors and enzymes associated with allergic rhinitis. *Phytother Res. 2009 Jul*; 23(7):920–6. doi: 10.1002/ptr.2763. PMID: 19140159.

46   Nzeako, B C et al. "Antimicrobial activities of clove and thyme extracts." *Sultan Qaboos University medical journal vol. 6,1 (2006): 33–9*.

47   Terlizzi, Maria E et al. "UroPathogenic Escherichia coli (UPEC) Infections: Virulence Factors, Bladder Responses, Antibiotic, and Non-antibiotic Antimicrobial Strategies." *Frontiers in microbiology vol. 8 1566*. 15 Aug. 2017, doi: 10.3389/fmicb.2017.01566

48   Mohajeri, M Hasan et al. "The role of the microbiome for human health: from basic science to clinical applications." *European journal of nutrition vol. 57, Suppl 1 (2018): 1–14*. doi: 10.1007/s00394-018–1703–4

49   Benavente-Garcia O. et al. Antioxidant activity of phenolics extracted from Olea europaea L. leaves. *Food Chem. 2000;68:457–462*. [Google Scholar]

50   Valenzuela et al. Hydroxytyrosol prevents reduction in liver activity of Δ-5 and Δ-6 desaturases, oxidative stress, and depletion in long chain polyunsaturated fatty acid content in different tissues of high-fat diet fed mice. *Lipids in Health and Disease. April 2017*. DOI: 10.1186/s12944-017–0450–5

51   Alizadeh-Navaei R et al. Investigation of the effect of ginger on the lipid levels. A double blind controlled clinical trial. *Saudi Med J. 2008 Sep*; 29(9):1280–4. PMID: 18813412.

52   Mahboubi Mohaddese, Mahboubi Mona. Hepatoprotection by dandelion (Taraxacum officinale) and mechanisms (2020). *Asian Pacific Journal of Tropical Biomedicine. Volume: 10, Issue Number: 1, Page: 1–10*

53   Kondo T et al. Vinegar intake reduces body weight, body fat mass, and serum triglyceride levels in obese Japanese subjects. *Biosci Biotechnol Biochem. 2009 Aug*; 73(8):1837–43. doi: 10.1271/bbb.90231. Epub 2009 Aug 7. PMID: 19661687.7)

54   Weiskirchen, Ralf et al. "The hop constituent xanthohumol exhibits hepatoprotective effects

and inhibits the activation of hepatic stellate cells at different levels." *Frontiers in physiology vol. 6 140*. 6 May. 2015, doi: 10.3389/fphys.2015.00140

55  Clifford, Tom et al. "The potential benefits of red beetroot supplementation in health and disease." *Nutrients vol. 7,4 2801–22*. 14 Apr. 2015, doi: 10.3390/nu7042801

56  britishlivertrust.org.uk/wp-content/uploads/The-health-benefits-of-coffee-BLT-report-June-2016.pdf. As of 03/02/21

57  Cheney, G. "Rapid healing of peptic ulcers in patients receiving fresh cabbage juice." *California medicine vol. 70,1 (1949)*: 10–5.

58  Narnoliya, Lokesh Kumar et al. "The Phytochemical Composition, Biological Effects and Biotechnological Approaches to the Production of High-Value Essential Oil from Geranium." *Essential Oil Research: Trends in Biosynthesis, Analytics, Industrial Applications and Biotechnological Production 327–352*. 9 Mar. 2019, doi: 10.1007/978–3–030–16546–8_12

59  Shinohara K, Doi H, Kumagai C, Sawano E, Tarumi W. Effects of essential oil exposure on salivary estrogen concentration in perimenopausal women. *Neuro Endocrinol Lett. 2017 Jan;37(8)*: 567–572. PMID: 28326753.

60  Khadivzadeh, Talat et al. "Effect of Fennel on the Health Status of Menopausal Women: A Systematic and Meta-analysis." *Journal of menopausal medicine vol. 24,1 (2018)*: 67–74. doi: 10.6118/jmm.2018.24.1.67

61  Narnoliya, Lokesh Kumar et al. "The Phytochemical Composition, Biological Effects and Biotechnological Approaches to the Production of High-Value Essential Oil from Geranium." *Essential Oil Research: Trends in Biosynthesis, Analytics, Industrial Applications and Biotechnological Production 327–352*. 9 Mar. 2019, doi: 10.1007/978–3–030–16546–8_12

62  www.ema.europa.eu/en/documents/herbal-report/draft-assessment-report-epilobium-angustifolium-l/epilobium-parviflorum-schreb-herba_en.pdf. As of 04/02/21.

63  Ghorbanibirgani, Alireza et al. "The efficacy of stinging nettle (urtica dioica) in patients with benign prostatic hyperplasia: a randomized double-blind study in 100 patients." *Iranian Red Crescent medical journal vol. 15,1 (2013)*: 9–10. doi: 10.5812/ircmj.2386

64  Safarinejad MR. Urtica dioica for treatment of benign prostatic hyperplasia: a prospective, randomized, double-blind, placebo-controlled, crossover study. *J Herb Pharmacother. 2005; 5(4)*: 1–11. PMID: 16635963.

65  Eleazu, Chinedum et al. "Management of Benign Prostatic Hyperplasia: Could Dietary Polyphenols Be an Alternative to Existing Therapies?." *Frontiers in pharmacology vol. 8 234*. 28 Apr. 2017, doi: 10.3389/fphar.2017.00234

66  Christensen R, Bartels EM, Altman RD et al. Does the hip powder of Rosa canina (rosehip) reduce pain in osteoarthritis patients? – a meta-analysis of randomized controlled trials. *Osteoarthritis Cartilage 2008; 16*: 965–972.

67  Rosenthal, Ann K. "Crystals, inflammation, and osteoarthritis." *Current opinion in rheumatology vol. 23,2 (2011)*: 170–3. doi: 10.1097/BOR.0b013e3283432d1f

68  Pareek, Anil et al. "Feverfew (Tanacetum parthenium L.): A systematic review." *Pharmacognosy reviews vol. 5,9 (2011)*: 103–10. doi: 10.4103/0973–7847.79105

69  Oral NaHCO3 Activates a Splenic Anti-Inflammatory Pathway: Evidence That Cholinergic Signals Are Transmitted via Mesothelial Cells. Sarah C. Ray, Babak Baban, Matthew A. Tucker, et al. *The Journal of Immunology April 16, 2018*, ji1701605; DOI: 10.4049/jimmunol.1701605

70  Medical College of Georgia at Augusta University. "Drinking baking soda could be an inexpensive, safe way to combat autoimmune disease." *ScienceDaily, 25 April 2018*. <www.sciencedaily.com/releases/2018/04/180425093745.htm>.

71  Sesterhenn K, Distl M, Wink M. Occurrence of iridoid glycosides in in vitro cultures and intact

plants of Scrophularia nodosa L. *Plant Cell Rep. 2007 Mar*; 26(3):365–71. doi: 10.1007/s00299–006–0233–3. Epub 2006 Sep 14. PMID: 16972093.

72   Jiang X, Qu Q, Li M, Miao S, Li X, Cai W. Horsetail mixture on rheumatoid arthritis and its regulation on TNF-α and IL-10. *Pak J Pharm Sci. 2014 Nov*;27(6 Suppl): 2019–23. PMID: 25410066.

73   Farinon, Mirian et al. "Effect of Aqueous Extract of Giant Horsetail (Equisetum giganteum L.) in Antigen-Induced Arthritis." *The open rheumatology journal vol. 7 129–33. 30 Dec. 2013*, doi: 10.2174/1874312901307010129

74   Jiang X, Qu Q, Li M, Miao S, Li X, Cai W. Horsetail mixture on rheumatoid arthritis and its regulation on TNF-α and IL-10. *Pak J Pharm Sci. 2014 Nov*; 27 (6 Suppl): 2019–23. PMID: 25410066.

75   Marstrand K, Campbell-Tofte J. The role of rose hip (Rosa canina L) powder in alleviating arthritis pain and inflammation – part II animal and human studies. *Botanics: Targets and Therapy. 2016*; 6:59–73, doi.org/10.2147/BTAT.S55573

76   Goutweed (Aegopodium podagraria L.) – botanical characteristics and prohealthy properties* Podagrycznik pospolity (Aegopodium podagraria L.) – charakterystyka botaniczna i właściwości prozdrowotne Karolina Jakubczyk1 , KatarzynaJanda1 ,Daniel Styburski2 , Agnieszka Łukomska3

77   Collins, Marcum W et al. "Is there a role for cherries in the management of gout?." *Therapeutic advances in musculoskeletal disease vol. 11 1759720X19847018. 17 May. 2019*, doi: 10.1177/1759720X19847018

78   digital.nhs.uk/news-and-events/news-archive/2017-news-archive/antidepressants-were-the-area-with-largest-increase-in-prescription-items-in-2016. As of 04/02/12

79   Iacobucci G. NHS prescribed record number of antidepressants last year. *BMJ. 2019 Mar 29*; 364:l1508. doi: 10.1136/bmj.l1508. PMID: 30926584.

80   H. Woelk, S. Schläfke, A multi-center, double-blind, randomised study of the Lavender oil preparation Silexan in comparison to Lorazepam for generalized anxiety disorder, *Phytomedicine, Volume 17, Issue 2, 2010*, Pages 94–99.

81   Kasper S, Müller WE, Volz HP, Möller HJ, Koch E, Dienel A. Silexan in anxiety disorders: Clinical data and pharmacological background. *World J Biol Psychiatry. 2018 Sep*; 19(6): 412–420. doi: 10.1080/15622975.2017.1331046. Epub 2017 Jun 19. PMID: 28511598.

82   J. Lehrner, G. Marwinski, S. Lehr, P. Johren, L. Deecke, Ambient odors of orange and lavender reduce anxiety and improve mood in a dental office, *Physiology & Behavior, Volume 86, Issues 1–2, 2005, Pages 92–95*.

# INDEX